IMAGE INTERPRETATION:
BONES, JOINTS, AND FRACTURES

IMAGE INTERPRETATION:
BONES, JOINTS, AND FRACTURES

James Harcus BHSc(Hons) MSc PgCert PgCHE FHEA
Lecturer in Diagnostic Imaging, School of Medicine
University of Leeds, United Kingdom

Voyin Pantic DCR (R) MSc PG Cert FETC
Lecturer, School of Medicine
University of Leeds, United Kingdom

For additional online content visit https://evolve.elsevier.com/cs/

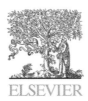

ELSEVIER

Content Strategist: Trinity Hutton; Clodagh Holland-Borosh
Content Project Manager: Ayan Dhar

Printed in Manipal Technologies Limited

Last digit is the print number: 9 8 7 6 5 4 3 2 1

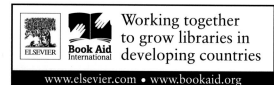

PREFACE

Image analysis and interpretation is a fundamental part of the role of a number of healthcare professionals. The ability to distinguish between normal and abnormal appearances and communicate findings is widely considered within the fundamental remit of diagnostic radiographers in many countries, where it is considered part of their role as part of their professional and regulatory standards.

For those beginning their education in image interpretation, it can be a very daunting and confusing experience. Trying to grasp the fundamental principles, normal anatomy, and pathologies can be overwhelming and it takes a combination of education and experience to develop proficiency in image interpretation.

One of the key things we teach at the start of a student's education in image interpretation is that a systematic and methodical approach to reviewing images is vital. Having a consistent way of reviewing medical images in the same way each time will help develop a framework of reference, building confidence and limiting missed abnormalities.

But how do you develop this systematic approach? This new text aims to provide an approach to radiographic images of the skeleton in relation to assessing normal anatomy of the skeleton and interpreting fractures and joint trauma by applying a systematic, methodical, step-by-step approach to radiographic images of the musculoskeletal system.

We recognise that radiographic image interpretation requires the understanding of numerous factors including radiographic technique and principles, as well as anatomy. The intention of this book, with its companion text *Bones and Joints, a guide for students*, is not to provide an exhaustive resource but to provide a succinct guide which can be used in four main ways:

1. To support a programme of study by covering the key principles of image interpretation and a systematic approach to radiographic images of the musculoskeletal system

2. For revision purposes, the accompanying online resources help to support the content in the book when preparing for image interpretation assessments

3. As a reference book and source of information for both the student and graduate health professional. The systematic approaches for each radiographic projection can be used directly in practical learning settings and the clinical environment

4. To form the basis for the student and graduate health professional to be able to take the information covered here and synthesise and apply it to new situations and scenarios

Chapters 1, 2, and 3 introduce some of the fundamental principles of reviewing radiographic images, understanding normal appearances, the need for a systematic approach, and an overview of fractures and joint injuries. Chapters 4–9 cover the different parts of the musculoskeletal system, providing an overview of what to assess, offering a structured approach for each radiographic image, and an overview of common and important fractures and trauma of the musculoskeletal system. Chapter 10 considers the role of the health professional in the communication of findings.

Despite the relatively succinct nature of the content, there is a lot of information, so where there are important or commonly misunderstood concepts, the 'Insights' within each chapter aim to highlight and further explain some of these.

ACKNOWLEDGEMENTS

Love and thanks go to Helen, Millie, and my family and friends for your ongoing support and patience. Thank you also to my colleague, co-author, and friend Voyin Pantic for supporting me since I was a student radiographer. He was the original reason I pursued image interpretation and education as a passion.

James Harcus
Lecturer in Diagnostic Imaging
University of Leeds

I would like to thank Caroline, William, Henri, and my family and friends for their continued support. In particular, I would like to thank my co-author and friend, James Harcus, who was a student of mine and whom I am now proud to call a colleague. As a lecturer, I am in a privileged position to have an impact on students, learn from them, and watch them flourish as professionals. My interest in image interpretation developed as a student and grew with my involvement with the first radiographer image interpretation course at the University of Leeds. Through many years, I developed the theme of image interpretation in the undergraduate programme at the University of Leeds.

Voyin Pantic
Lecturer in Diagnostic Imaging
University of Leeds

CONTENTS

PRINCIPLES OF IMAGE INTERPRETATION

1

INTRODUCTION

This chapter will explore general principles of image interpretation which act as a foundation on which to build. Image interpretation is a complex subject and is idiosyncratic in nature. This whole text will introduce systematic approaches and aspects to consider when viewing radiographic images. It has been well documented that understanding through education improves an individual's ability to distinguish between normal and abnormal appearances. No one approach addresses an individual's needs and as such this text provides the basis on which to build and develop your skills in the area of image interpretation.

KEY ASPECTS OF IMAGE INTERPRETATION

Four key requirements have been identified which can be applied to all radiographic image interpretation, one of these being *an understanding of what is in the image*. This can be applied to an understanding of the physical principles of how the image is produced. An appreciation of the reasons for the presentation of the various shades on the image as well as how altering the image parameters affects these and other aspects of the resultant image is required. A full discussion of these factors is beyond the scope of this text.

Another key requirement is to *understand what the patient is*. An understanding of the anatomy, relationships and anatomical features, normal variations, and pathological and injury presentations is essential. Understanding where anatomical features are enables the observer to appreciate where they will be located on an image and how they appear.

INSIGHT

The clinical details the patient presents with will inform the observer as to why the investigation is necessary and potentially what appearances are likely to be present. But beware that you do not focus on the area directed by the clinical details alone but review the full image to ensure that no aspect is overlooked.

In order to fully appreciate the appearance contained within the radiographic image, the observer needs to *understand what was conducted*. In planar X-ray imaging standardisation is key. By producing standard radiographic images the observer is able to develop a framework of reference, which enables them to use their mentally stored data set of radiographic image appearances to compare the image to; this can be likened to a mental version of spot the difference. Any deviation from the standard projection needs to be identified in order that this can be considered when reviewing the radiographic image and reduce the potential for misinterpretation.

 INSIGHT

An example of this would be undertaking a lateral knee using a horizontal beam. The use of legends to indicate the deviation from norm allows the observer to take this into account when reviewing the radiographic image and thus attributing any changes to this fact.

Finally *be aware of the limitations of the procedure*. In planar X-ray imaging the resultant radiographic image can be considered to be formed by a process of summation of shadows. Simply put, the overlying anatomical structure will attenuate the X-ray beam to various amounts. The multiple overlying shadows can be difficult to interpret due to the presence of multiple lines. In addition to this, an awareness of the spatial resolution of the imaging modality used is essential in determining whether this is the reason that features are currently not visualized, as it is beyond the current resolution capabilities for that image modality.

 INSIGHT

A fractured scaphoid or pathology may have changes that are too subtle to be resolved by planar X-ray imaging, and thus the radiographic image has a normal appearance when there is an abnormality present. In both cases follow-up examinations or other clinical tests are required in order to identify whether there is an abnormality present.

These principles can be utilised when reviewing any image. The identification of individual carpal bones on a lateral wrist is complex due to the overlapping nature of a three-dimensional structure being represented as a two-dimensional structure. Review Fig. 1.1, a radiographic image of a normal lateral wrist.

Fig. 1.1 Radiograph of a lateral wrist. (Source: Alphonsus K.S. Chong, Jin Xi Lim, David M.K. Tan. Diagnostic Imaging of the Hand and Wrist, 2018.)

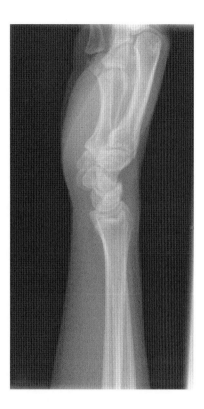

By understanding what is in the image we can appreciate that there are areas that appear radiopaque (brighter) and those that appear radiolucent (darker). Through understanding these aspects we can appreciate that for areas to appear radiopaque there has to be greater attenuation of the X-ray beam and therefore greater bone density. This can be used to identify where bones are superimposed.

Understanding what is in the patient can assist in identifying individual carpal bones. For example, we know that there are eight carpal bones. We know that the carpal bones are divided up into two rows (proximal and distal). We can utilise the shapes and relationships of the carpal bones to further aid us in recognising individual carpal bones. Applying this to the image the lunate can be recognised due to its distinctive crescent shape and appreciating that it is located in the proximal row, and its relationship with the distal aspect of the radius. Relationship can also be used to identify the capitate, which is located with the cup of the lunate and is also the largest carpal bone.

Understanding what was conducted is also essential; understanding the position of the patient and the direction of the X-ray beam allows us to orientate ourselves with the image, in addition to our familiarity with the shape of the structure. By identifying the anterior and posterior aspects and understanding which structures are more anterior, this can be applied to identify more carpal bones.

Putting together the facts so far, we can see a carpal bone that is present anteriorly; this carpal bone is radiolucent anteriorly and is superimposed on another carpal bone, which gives it a radiopaque appearance posteriorly. Following the margin of this carpal bone it can be seen that it is round and can be identified as the pisiform.

Identifying the first metacarpal bone of the thumb by appreciating that this bone is shorter than the other metacarpals and broader enables us to identify the trapezium through understanding relationships. Furthermore, there is a radiopacity adjacent to the trapezium at the distal aspect of the capitate, which represents the trapezoid in the distal row of carpal bones. In the proximal row of the carpal bones there is a radiopacity associated with the pisiform, which can be identified as the triquetral.

The distinctive shape of the scaphoid and its location in the proximal row and relationships with the trapezium and lunate allow us to identify this carpal bone.

The limitation of this image having multiple overlying shadows makes it extremely difficult to identify the hamate. Aspects of the hamate can be identified through the association of lines that are not related to any of the other carpal bones.

 INSIGHT

As can be seen, appreciating these factors is the first step on the journey of image interpretation.

 EXERCISE

Compare the following two Cartoon skeleton 1 and Cartoon skeleton 2 (Figs. 1.2 and 1.3) and identify the difference between them. When comparing the difference, consider which ones are spotted first and how long it takes you to spot the differences.

Although the cartoon skeleton is a simplified version, there is familiarity, so the appearance is not alien to you. From studying anatomy you recognise what anatomical features are represented and as such understand what is in the patient. You have more than likely undertaken spot-the-difference activities and are familiar with what needs to be conducted and have developed an approach to undertaking this activity. The limitations could be a number of factors; you have no context in that you do not know how many differences you are looking for, and others could include finding the exercise simplistic and not paying full attention to this or external disturbances affecting full concentration. Having two images helps in image interpretation and this is the main reason to review whether your patient has any previous relevant images in order for you to compare any changes.

Fig. 1.2 Cartoon skeleton 1, and Fig. 1.3 Cartoon skeleton 2.

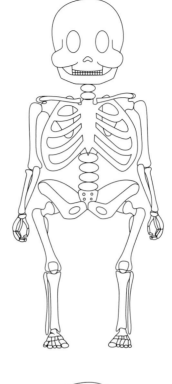

Fig. 1.3 Cartoon skeleton 2.

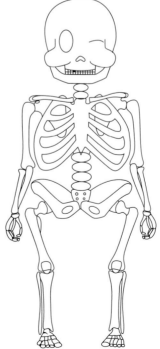

The differences can be found on page 13. It is recommended that you do not review these until you have completed this chapter.

The process you have just undertaken is one of information reduction. To achieve this successfully you will have applied some form of search pattern to ensure that you review all of the image and thus not omit any changes. Failure to apply this approach can lead to the phenomenon of *'satisfaction of search error'*. This error occurs when not all differences have been identified. In radiographic image interpretation this can occur when an abnormality is identified that answers the clinical question but a second abnormality present is overlooked. The satisfaction of search error occurs due to the image not being fully reviewed. In subsequent chapters in this book you will be introduced to systematic reviews, which should aid you in developing your image interpretation skills and provide you with aspects to consider in order to review the radiographic image fully.

Context

To assist with the exercise context can help. Context can be applied to the two images (Figs. 1.2 and 1.3) you have reviewed. Context is relevant information to aid you in fully understanding the information present – in this case to guide you to identify all the changes. As such, the additional information is that there are four differences between the two images. If you have not identified four differences, review the images again to see if you are able to spot them.

Review Fig. 1.4; the central figure can be perceived in one of two ways. If reading the horizontal line from left to right, the central figure is interpreted as a letter B, as the other horizontal figures are all recognised as letters, whereas if reading from top to bottom, the central figure becomes the number 13, which is consistent with the other figures in the vertical line.

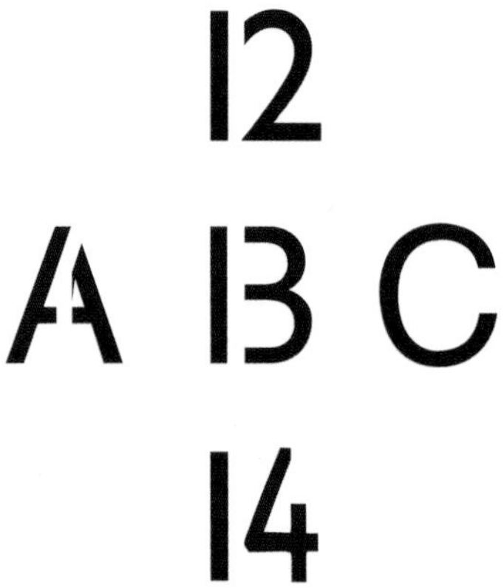

Fig. 1.4 How perception is influenced by context. (Source: Wine Tasting: A Professional Handbook, Third Edition, 2017.)

INSIGHT

Context can have an impact on visual perception. Therefore it is essential that we ensure that the clinical details we are presented with are accurate to ensure that we are not misled when reviewing the image.

Familiarity

Familiarity is essential to image interpretation. If we do not know what we are looking at, then the object being observed has no meaning to us and therefore cannot be recognised. Or we assign a meaning by projecting our expectations onto the image which fits with our understanding of the world.

Fig. 1.5 may appear as random series of black-and-white patterns. Through closer observation the patterns may form recognisable shapes. Words can be used to help us recognise and interpret the image. If 'dog' was given as a clue, then as an observer we would be looking for familiar patterns that match that of a dog. Further contextualisation could further help in the interpretation of the image, for example, 'the dog is sniffing the ground'.

Once the image is recognised, we have a sense of closure, the 'ah ha!' moment when everything becomes clear. Up until that point there was a sense of frustration in the lack of ability to make sense of the patterns.

Just as in Fig. 1.5, we are seeking patterns that match objects which are familiar to us. This image has been inverted, and this may make the pattern less obvious. Fig. 1.6 is a photograph taken of the surface of Mars; do you notice anything familiar in the photograph? Review the whole image in a systematic way seeking patterns that might be familiar to you. Review Fig. 1.7: is there any feature more obvious. When we make observations, eye movements (saccades) are subconscious. The eyes will fixate on points of interest. Yarbus (1967) used pictures of faces to track eye movement. It was noted that eyes fixed over

Fig. 1.5 Series of black-and-white patterns. (Source: Wine Tasting: A Professional Handbook, Third Edition, 2017.)

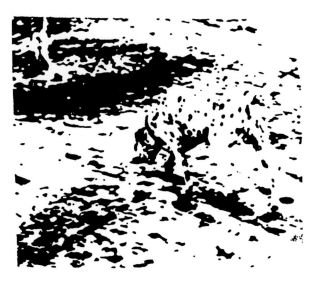

Fig. 1.6 1976 NASA photograph of the surface of Mars. (Source: Shaul Hochstein, Orit Hershler. With a careful look: Still no low-level confound to face pop-out, 2006.)

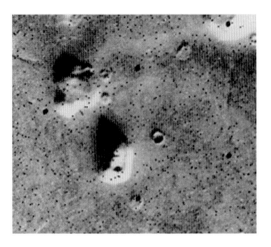

certain points these being the eyes, nose and mouth, as well as the outline of the head. All these features are present in Fig. 1.6 and Fig. 1.7, leading our brain to interpret these patterns as a head. It is important to ensure that we observe the whole image and not fixate on the obvious in order to avoid the phenomenon of satisfaction of search.

Consider Figs. 1.8 and 1.9 to identify what they represent. Is one easier to identify than the other?

Fig. 1.7 1976 NASA photograph known as "the Face on Mars." (Source: Shaul Hochstein, Orit Hershler. With a careful look: Still no low-level confound to face pop-out, 2006.)

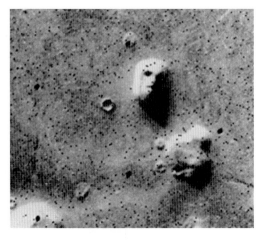

In Fig. 1.8 there is recognisable anatomy that we are familiar with, as well as less familiar anatomy in terms of shapes. Through knowledge of anatomy even features of unfamiliar anatomy can be recognised. The utilisation of previous knowledge can be applied to the current image to make sense of what is being viewed. For example, you are aware of what a human chest radiographic image looks like, and that this image does not appear to be human.

Fig. 1.9 is much more difficult to interpret, as the appearance is more than likely alien to you due to a lack of familiarity. There are some radiolucencies and radiopacities, which you could assume are air filled and bone, respectively. The

Fig. 1.8 What do you recognise? (Source: Sara M. Gardhouse, David Eshar. Ferrets, Rabbits, and Rodents: Clinical Medicine and Surgery, Fourth Edition, 2021.)

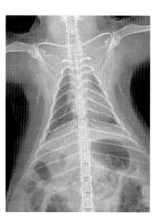

Fig. 1.9 What do you recognise? (Source: Joseph P. Fowler's Zoo and Wild Animal Medicine, 2015.)

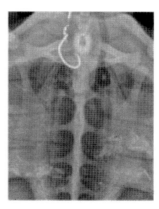

central radiopaque structure you could assume was the spine due to its position and some features. In this image the big clue is the artefact present, which looks like a fishhook and gives a clue as to the habitat that this creature occupies.

 INSIGHT

When drawing conclusions only use evidence that you can justify. This process can be termed a *detective model* where the conclusion is evidence based.

As can be seen from the evidence presented, certain conclusions can be reached. For another conclusion to be reached, more evidence/information is required. In this case a conclusion cannot be reached as to what animal the image represents; this is not too dissimilar to radiographic imaging. Some abnormalities present with similar appearances, and with certainty it can be identified that the patient has an abnormality, but it is not always possible to identify precisely what the abnormality is without further investigations, which may or may not be imaging.

Fig. 1.8 was that of a mammal, a prairie dog, as seen in Fig. 1.10. Fig. 1.9 was that of a reptile, a turtle, as seen in Fig. 1.11. The visualisation of the full image

Fig. 1.10 Prairie dog. (Source: Ferrets, Rabbits, and Rodents: Clinical Medicine and Surgery, Fourth Edition, 2021.)

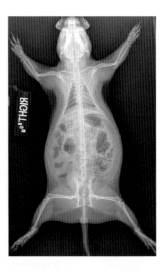

Fig. 1.11 Turtle. (Source: Fowler's Zoo and Wild Animal Medicine, 2015.)

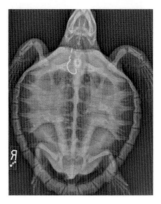

allows us to recognise the animals, as you are familiar with their appearances. The anatomy of the prairie dog is more familiar to you than that of the turtle, and hence easier to recognise what it represents.

FRAMEWORK OF REFERENCE

In order to appreciate abnormal appearances it is essential to appreciate how the normal state is presented in an image. For the purpose of this chapter Fig. 1.2 will be used to represent the normal state. By implication, all the changes identified on Fig. 1.3 can be considered as representing abnormal changes. This can be considered as developing a framework of reference for this image. In this case you are formulating a mental construct of what is normal by using Fig. 1.2. The mental construct or framework will be one that you will use to compare other images to, just as was done in the exercise to determine whether there are any deviations from normal. The mental construct is vital, as this will be used as your framework of reference in the case when there are no images to compare against. This is more challenging than a simple spot-the-difference, as you are relying on information that has been internalised on which to base your opinion as to whether the image is considered normal or not; in other words, you will not always have a 'normal' radiographic image to compare to.

Standardisation

Standardisation is a key aspect in developing a framework of reference. Through applying standard techniques to produce medical images of various anatomy the observer is able to develop a framework of reference in order to compare one image with another, be that physically through comparing to previous radiographic images the patient has had or mentally through previous experiences and knowledge gained from viewing and understanding appearances from many radiographic images of the area currently being reviewed. Deviation from standard techniques leads to the introduction of variables that the observer may or may not be familiar with, which limits the effectiveness of being able to interpret the image. As identified, familiarity is key to image interpretation.

If we consider Fig. 1.12, this figure could demonstrate a radiographic image of a cube. If this was the case, then there are two possible positions of the cube that would result in the production of this image as identified in Fig. 1.13, with the two leading edges of each cube identified, one by the green line and the other by the red. If this was a clinical examination, it would be important to know which position was used to obtain the radiographic image for accurate interpretation. To overcome this problem, an agreement as to the standard positioning of the cube could be reached to be able to accurately interpret the image.

 INSIGHT

This is why it is essential in clinical practice to annotate the images if non-standardised practice is used to produce an image. This ensures that the observers of the image can take the non-standardised practice into consideration during interpretation.

When competing information, as in Fig. 1.12, is present, this is known as dissonance. Another example of dissonance is E. G Boring's image of the Old

Fig. 1.12 Line drawing of a cube.

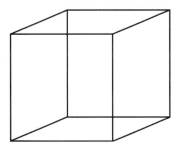

Fig. 1.13 Line drawing of a cube with leading edges identified for the two different cubes, one red and the other green. (Source: Moran Furman. Neuronal Networks in Brain Function, CNS Disorders, and Therapeutics, 2014)

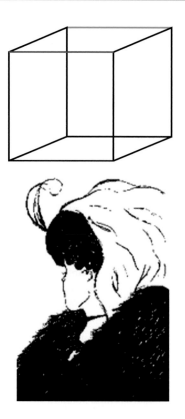

Fig. 1.14 Old or Young Woman. (Source: My Wife and My Mother-In-Law, by the cartoonist W. E. Hill, 1915 (adapted from a picture going back at least to a 1888 German postcard).)

and Young woman (Fig. 1.14.) The constants for both images are the fur coat, the feather in the hair, the hair, and the head covering. The young woman is looking away from the reader, over her shoulder, whereas the old woman's nose is represented by the chin and the angle of the mandible of the young woman. The young woman's ear becomes the old woman's eye. The choker of the young woman is the old woman's mouth.

What is the first thing you see when viewing Fig. 1.15?

Fig. 1.15 "All Is Vanity" by Charles Allan Gilbert (1892). (Source: Michael Cohen Jr. Orthognathic Surgery: Principles and Practice, Oxford University Press, 2014.)

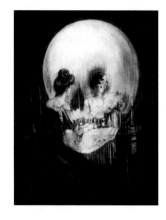

At first glance you may interpret Fig. 1.15 as a skull. Upon closer inspection you see a different picture emerging of a woman sitting at a dressing table. It is essential that we are able to concentrate on the image in order to make the correct interpretation and not a rash decision.

Words

Precise and accurate description is required in image interpretation. It is important that the individual who reads your description is able to understand and accurately locate what you are describing. There should be little room for ambiguity in your description as to where any changes occur.

EXERCISE

Refer back to page 5, Fig. 1.3. Write down as precisely as you can where the differences are in Fig. 1.3. Reproduce Fig. 1.2 and give it to a colleague along with your description. Ask your colleague to draw on the image where the areas are identified in your description. How accurately did the colleague identify the changes on the image?
  Were some easier to describe than others?
  Consider which were easier and why. How could your description have been improved?

EXERCISE. ANSWERS

You were provided with misleading information in the context. Did you spot that there was an extra difference? Did you miss it?
  The five differences are: winking left eye; black/missing right upper tooth; medial/vertebral border of scapula missing; left lesser trochanter missing; right distal missing phalanx of the little toe.

NORMALISING

One of the features that could have been overlooked is the missing scapula line. Even though the line is not present, the brain inserts information to account for the anomaly; this is an example of normalising.

INSIGHT

The context was misleading, as it gave the incorrect number of differences. If you identified four differences, you would have considered the exercise complete. As previously identified, this is related to satisfaction of search; you were satisfied that you had identified all the differences. If you had carried on, then you may have identified the additional difference. Do not be misled by information; make sure that you continue your search of the image even if you have detected the change consistent with the clinical details, just in case there are more anomalies.

SUMMARY

The following diagrammatic presentation (Fig. 1.16) by Anook van der Gijp et al. (2015) provides a summary of the factors considered in this chapter as well as brings in aspects that will be covered in other chapters in this book. A key aspect identified in the synthesis circle is 'deciding about advice and action'. This can be translated into recognising and reflecting on your own limitation so that you are aware of which areas need to be developed.

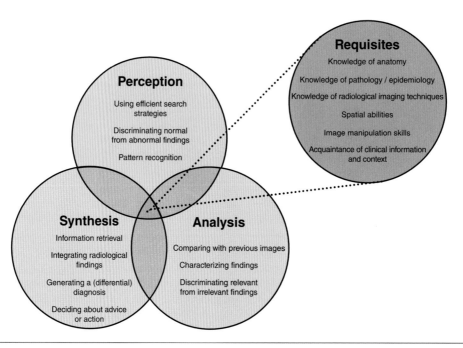

Fig. 1.16 Attributes contributing to image interpretation. (Source: van der Gijp A, et al: Volumetric and two-dimensional image interpretation show different cognitive processes in learners, Acad Radiol 22(5):632–639, 2015.)

Further Reading

van der Gijp, A., et al. (2015). Volumetric and two-dimensional image interpretation show different cognitive processes in learners. *Academic Radiology, 22*(5), 632–639.

Gary, L., Rahman, R. A., Boroditsky, L., & Clark, A. (2020). Effects of language on visual perception. *Trends in Cognitive Sciences, 24*(11), 930–944.

Robinson, P. J. A. (1996). The nature of image reporting. In A. Patterson & R. Price (Eds.), *Current topics in radiography* (2nd ed.). W B Saunders Company Ltd.

Yarbus, A. L. (2021). *Eye movements and vision*. New York: Plenum Press.

NORMAL APPEARANCES – A SYSTEMIC APPROACH

2

When we review any medical image, as discussed in Chapter 1, it is imperative that we do so in a methodical and systematic way. This ensures that we have reviewed and assessed all of the information available to us and have given ourselves the best opportunity to identify all potential abnormalities within it. This is known as *satisfaction of search* – we are satisfied we have searched the entire image and are satisfied we have not missed anything.

When we evaluate an image with an obvious abnormality on it, we tend to focus on this first. This is known as salience, and if we allow it to distract our attention, then we may overlook other important findings. So we have to try and ignore it, review the rest of the image, and then come back to it.

In order to do this so that we become more proficient, and ultimately quicker, at image interpretation, it is best to approach the evaluation of images in a systematic way. This will help you move around the image methodically, review all of the necessary information, and hopefully identify any abnormalities (or be confident it is normal).

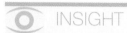 INSIGHT

When reviewing radiological images, it is important to apply a *systematic approach* and to scrutinise all parts of the images through a '*satisfaction of search*' to avoid missing abnormalities. If one abnormality is identified, look for more (Fig. 2.1).

Force yourself to go through these systematic approaches. It takes time and effort at first, but by reviewing images in the same way every time and practising, you will become quicker, more confident, and less likely to overlook any aspect!

Fig. 2.1 How many fractures? This right shoulder demonstrates multiple rib fractures (arrows). Without a systematic approach and satisfaction of search, the distal clavicle fracture (hollow arrow) may well have been overlooked. (Source: Diagnostic Imaging: Chest, STATdx © Elsevier.)

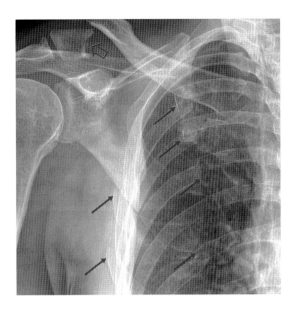

When evaluating a medical image, regardless of what the image is, STOP! Go through the image in a systematic way, make a note of the significant findings as you go, then come back to them once you are happy you have reviewed the entire image.

Often with complex findings, there are lots of pieces of information which you can collect and put together to come up with the answer, or diagnosis. It is a bit like a jigsaw puzzle; you need all of the pieces. A systematic approach helps us to collect those pieces to reveal the final answer!

The aim of this book is to improve skeletal image interpretation skills, and a systematic approach is essential to this. In this chapter we consider some of the generic aspects of a systematic approach which, in the subsequent chapters, can be applied to specific images of the bones and joints.

Before we start thinking about looking for abnormalities, however, we have to consider what normal bones and joints look like on radiographic images.

NORMAL RADIOGRAPHIC APPEARANCES

Radiographic images are made up of a range of different shades (or brightness) of grey, from black to white and an infinite number of shades in between (though the human eye cannot differentiate all of them). The brightness demonstrated on the image is directly related to how much the X-ray beam is *attenuated* (or absorbed/scattered) within the patient.

The denser and thicker the tissues, the more of the X-ray beam is attenuated and the more radiopaque (brighter/whiter) it will appear; cortical bone, for example, appears densely radiopaque (brighter), cancellous bone less radiopaque (darker), and soft tissues even less so. Air appears very radiolucent (black), since it attenuates virtually none of the X-ray beam.

Normal and abnormal tissues appear the way they do on radiographs because of the degree of attenuation of the X-ray beam as it passes through them and is captured on the image receptor. It is therefore important when interpreting images that you understand the interaction processes that result in the final image (as covered in Chapter 1).

When we look at spotting abnormalities, such as fractures, we can use this to help explain what we see. In a simplified way, abnormalities may appear:

- *Too radiopaque* (sclerotic in the case of bone); denser (whiter/brighter) than we would normally expect
- *Too radiolucent* (lytic in the case of bone); less dense (blacker/darker) than we would normally expect
- *Too large*; bigger than we would normally expect
- *Too small*
- *Missing/displaced;* not evident or moved away from their normal position

It is important first of all that you understand what normal appearances look like so that you have a clear framework of reference by which it becomes easier to identify when things are abnormal. In the next section we will look at the normal appearances of bones and joints by using a systematic approach which we can apply and use, regardless of what body part we are looking at.

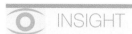

INSIGHT

'Before you can know what is abnormal, you must first know what is normal.'

Identifying abnormalities on images relies on us knowing what 'normal' is supposed to look like. Understanding the normal appearances, including those related to age and normal variants, gives us a reference point to then spot when things are abnormal. Having a good understanding of the anatomy and 'normal' images helps to build this appreciation of normal.

A SYSTEMATIC APPROACH – AABCSS

There are numerous different approaches which can be used when assessing radiographic images; the ABCS (alignment, bones, cartilage, soft tissues) approach is one of the more commonly utilised, particularly because it is simple to follow!

What it requires is that you follow each of the steps to look at the entire image in terms of each bone, joint, and soft tissue feature for the image.

What is perhaps missing in this approach are two key factors: assessment of image quality (very important in image interpretation) and reviewing specific important areas which may commonly be missed or where significant injuries may occur; we call these review areas.

So, throughout the rest of this book we will use the following systematic approach when reviewing the radiographic images using AABCSS:

A	Adequacy	assess the image quality of the image
A	Alignment	do the bones/joints maintain normal shape and alignment?
B	Bones	is there any evidence of fracture/pathology in the individual bones?
C	Cartilage	specifically this asks you to look at the joint spaces (i.e. where the cartilage is)
S	Soft Tissues	assess the soft tissue structures and lines
S	Significant Areas	looking at review areas for commonly missed/significant pathology

The approach will vary according to the part of the body being imaged, but we will now consider some general principles when looking at radiographic images of bones and joints.

We recommend refreshing your knowledge of bone structure, growth, and appearances before reading the rest of this chapter, if you are unsure of any of these aspects.

A – Adequacy

An area that may well be forgotten when we consider image interpretation is actually considering whether the quality of the image being reviewed is technically adequate. Many of the appearances, concepts, lines, and signs we use to help us determine whether an image is normal or not depend on the image being of an adequate quality according to recognised standards.

Sub-optimal-quality images may mimic or hide abnormalities, so our confidence in whether an image is normal or not should be determined by the quality of the image; a high-quality image gives us more confidence in our decision.

Whilst we strive for all medical images to be of optimal image quality (whilst maintaining the *as low as reasonably practicable* – ALARP – principle), in practice, this is not always possible, particularly in trauma or where the patient's condition will not allow. In assessing image quality, though, we can identify sub-optimal quality and allow for it when we are assessing for abnormality.

This means that the first part of any image review should be to assess the image quality, or *adequacy*, of the images being reviewed. As previously discussed, we should do this in a systematic way, and there are many described checklists available for assessing adequacy; like other systematic approaches, the more it is used, the quicker and easier it becomes to do. It is outside the scope of this text to consider all aspects of image quality in detail; instead, we will summarise the key aspects to review:

Patient demographics – is this the correct patient, is the examination the most current one (even in teaching cases where this is not present, get into the habit of checking these aspects)?

Anatomical marker – check for its presence and that it appears correct; for example, is the left ankle labelled as the left?

Area of interest – what body part has been imaged, has everything been included that is required, has anything been excluded that needs to be?

Projections/Positioning – what radiographic projections have been taken, are they positioned adequately?

Exposure – assessment of exposure factors such as resolution and contrast; can we see fine detail such as bone trabecular pattern? Can we visualise soft tissue planes as well as bony anatomy?

Artefacts – are there any artefacts on the image (either in or on the patient) which may be obscuring anatomy?

Repeats – would we need to repeat or try and improve any of the images based upon the previous points?

Pathology – are there any abnormalities/fractures/pathologies present? Note how the aspect of looking for abnormalities comes last on the list!!

 INSIGHT

When reviewing images, assessment of image adequacy should come first: is the image of diagnostic quality? Consideration of abnormalities should be second.

A – Alignment

Each bone has a 'normal' typical shape. Where bones meet at a joint, the articular surfaces of each bone meet to form congruence of the joint: its normal shape. Fractures and joint injuries can cause a displacement in this normal alignment (or shape) of a bone or joint.

- Look at each bone in turn; does it maintain its normal shape?
- Look at the joints on the image where the bones meet; are the articular surfaces of the bones still congruent (i.e. do they still align where they are supposed to)?

Many bones and joints have imaginary radiographic lines or angles associated with them which can be used to assess the congruity and alignment of them. These will be considered individually within each relevant chapter, but some examples include:

- *Anterior humeral line*: used to assess for displaced fractures in the distal humerus (Fig. 2.2)
- *Shenton's line*: associated with fractures of the femoral neck
- *Anterior vertebral line*: follows the anterior aspect of the vertebral bodies, may be disrupted in spinal injuries

If reviewing a long bone where two joints are included at each end, then assess the alignment between the two joints; are they grossly aligned (e.g. both AP/lateral depending on the projection)?

 INSIGHT

It is useful to learn the relevant radiographic lines when assessing alignment on an image; they may be a useful indicator of bone or soft tissue injury (which we might not otherwise visualise).

We do not often carry round protractors in our pockets to measure angles, but image review stations often contain software to measure them.

Fig. 2.2 Alignment; lateral left elbow. The anterior humeral line (dotted line) should normally bisect the middle third of the capitulum (C), as it does in **(A)**.

(B), in a paediatric patient, demonstrates the anterior humeral line does not pass through the middle of the capitulum indicating loss of normal alignment caused by a supracondylar fracture. The fracture is otherwise not visible. (Source: Diagnostic Imaging: Musculoskeletal Non-Trauma, STATdx © Elsevier.)

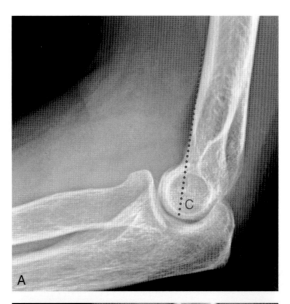

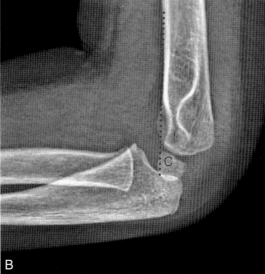

B – Bones

This aspect of the systematic approach perhaps takes the longest, as the bones typically form the majority of the information on a radiograph of the skeletal system and there may be many on an image, each of which has to be assessed in turn. The key is (again) to have a consistent systematic approach to how you look at them in turn (suggestions will be given in specific chapters).

When assessing bones on a radiograph, we have to first consider the underlying anatomy and how they appear radiographically (Fig. 2.3):

Fig. 2.3 Normal bone appearances; right ankle. (Source: Bontrager's Handbook of Radiographic Positioning and Techniques, Tenth Edition, 2021.)
A – Compact bone/cortex;
B – medullary cavity;
C – cancellous bone (trabeculae pattern visible);
D – fused epiphyseal plate remnant.

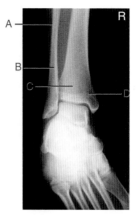

- *Cortex* – the peripheral outer layer of bone which is made up of dense compact bone made of regular units called osteons. Makes up the diaphysis (shaft) of long bones. Appears sclerotic (bright) on radiographs.
- *Cancellous bone* – found deep to compact bone at the ends of long bones and centre of other bones. Bone structure aligned under directions of stress into columns, called *trabeculae*. Less sclerotic/radiopaque than cortical bone.
- *Trabeculae* – individual structures which make up the cancellous bone, referred to as the trabecular pattern. Fine sclerotic lines demonstrated within cancellous bone. More prominent in some bones than others, for example, the proximal femur.
- *Medullary canal* – found within the centre of the diaphysis of long bones, contains yellow bone marrow predominantly. Appears more radiolucent than the peripheral compact bone.
- *Nutrient lines* – allow neurovascular structures to enter and leave the bone (don't forget, bone is a living tissue which needs a blood supply). In long bones these are normally found on one side of the cortex in the mid-diaphysis (shaft) and are typically orientated obliquely. They appear as ill-defined faint radiolucent lines in comparison with the density of the surrounding bone (Fig. 2.4).

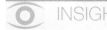 INSIGHT

Nutrient lines can sometimes be mistaken as a fracture because both appear as radiolucent lines within the bone. There are several key features to differentiate them (Fig. 2.4).

	Nutrient Line	Fracture
Appearance	Faint, ill-defined	More prominent, well-defined
Location	Usually in the mid-diaphysis	Can be anywhere
Orientation/shape	Oblique, linear	Can be in any direction/shape
Cortical step present?	No	Often

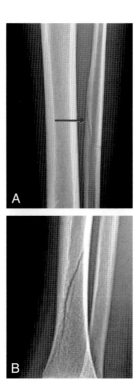

Fig. 2.4 Nutrient line (A). Note the appearances of the nutrient line (arrow) compared to the fracture of the tibia **(B)**. (Source: Diagnostic Imaging: Musculoskeletal Non-Trauma, STATdx © Elsevier.)

- *Sesamoid bones* – small bones found within tendons. Variable between individuals, the patella is the most common, but they are also found around other joints, particularly in the hands and feet. May be confused with avulsion fracture but will be round, be smooth, have a cortical margin, and not fit back onto the adjacent bone.

Bone appearances related to growth (Fig. 2.5) may be confused with fractures:

- *Epiphyseal (growth) plates* – site of growth in immature long bones. Found at either end between the metaphysis and epiphysis. Appear as a radiolucent line transversely across the bone. When fused in the mature skeleton, a remnant (Fig. 2.3) may often be seen demonstrated as a fine sclerotic line where the epiphyseal growth plate used to be.
- *Apophyses* – secondary sites of ossification, usually at the site of a bony protuberance. Appear as separate small pieces of bone until they fuse with skeletal maturity. Can be avulsed (pulled off) in trauma. Examples will be discussed in each chapter.
- *Hyaline cartilage model* (Fig. 2.6) – most bones in the skeleton are formed by intra-cartilaginous ossification. A hyaline cartilage model of the entire bone develops in utero, which then begins to ossify up to skeletal maturity. Radiographically only the ossified parts are visible; we cannot see the unossified cartilage but we need to remember it is still there, and this can fracture too.

Fig. 2.5 Normal bone appearances; paediatric left foot. (Source: Imaging Anatomy: Knee, Ankle, Foot, STATdx © Elsevier.)
A – Epiphysis;
B – epiphyseal plate;
C – apophysis (of base of 5th metatarsal);
D – sesamoid bone.

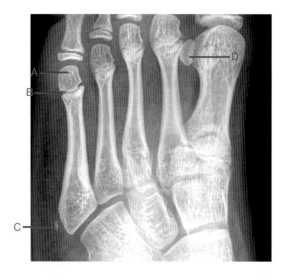

Fig. 2.6 Hyaline cartilage model; right wrist. Note the apparent 'missing' carpal bones in this 5-year-old **(A)** compared to a mature skeleton **(B)**. They are not missing; the cartilage model is present, just not ossified yet. Also note the subtle fractures (arrows) of the radius and ulna demonstrated only by a very subtle bulge or step in the cortex. (Source: Diagnostic Imaging: Pediatrics, STATdx © Elsevier.)

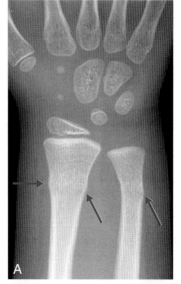

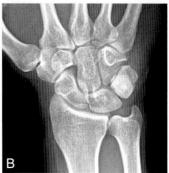

INSIGHT

Immature (not completely ossified) bone appears different to adult bone. They appear incomplete, and it appears there are more of them, or a part has been avulsed (pulled) off. It is important to remember paediatric bones are essentially the same shape as adult bones, just made in part of hyaline cartilage and therefore not always fully visible radiographically (Fig. 2.6).

When assessing bones, there are two main things we should consider:

- *Follow the cortex* – trace the periphery of the bone. Look for any interruptions in the smooth cortex which might indicate fracture, such as steps, lumps, or gaps (Fig. 2.6).
- *Assess the internal texture* – look for lucent fracture lines, look for sclerotic lines (where bone has been impacted on itself and appears more dense), and assess the trabecular pattern. In some bones, such as the proximal femur, the trabecular pattern appears very uniform and organised, so it is easier to see if disrupted (Fig. 2.7).

Fig. 2.7 Bones; subtle fracture; right neck of femur. There is a faint horizontal band of 'smudgy' sclerosis (arrow) and small step in the cortex (hollow arrow). Note the prominent trabecular pattern often seen in the proximal femur. (Source: Diagnostic Imaging: Musculoskeletal Trauma, STATdx © Elsevier.)

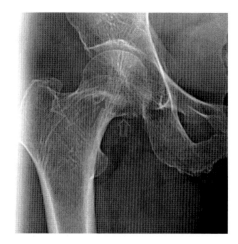

 INSIGHT

Due to the two-dimensional images produced of a three-dimensional structure, there will often be the superimposition of other structures over bones, such as other bones or soft tissue lines. These structures often look similar to fracture lines and can be misrepresented as such. This is known as the *Mach effect* (Fig. 2.8) and is a well-known phenomenon in image interpretation errors. A good appreciation of normal anatomy (again), understanding the relationship of different bones, and following the line in its entirety will help distinguish whether it is a fracture or not. If the line continues outside of the bone, then it can't be a fracture. Orthogonal (additional) projections are also helpful, if available.

Fig. 2.8 Mach effect; left foot. The soft tissue of the little toe mimics a fracture of the 4th toe proximal phalanx (arrow). (Source: Imaging Anatomy: Knee, Ankle, Foot, STATdx © Elsevier.)

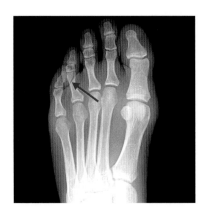

C – Cartilage

By this step, we mean we are assessing the joint spaces which are predominantly made up of cartilage (hyaline or fibro-) or fibrous tissue, dependent on the type of joint. In synovial joints there will also be a very small amount of synovial fluid.

We cannot normally see any of these tissues radiographically, but the width of the joint space gives a clue regarding the state of these tissues, and also the integrity of the joint following trauma.

- *Assess the width of the joint spaces* – are they widened or narrowed? Can be assessed alongside alignment.

The joint may appear widened if it has been 'pulled apart', which is known as diastasis.

Dislocations (Fig. 2.9) and subluxations may cause widening of a joint, as well as a loss of alignment, but sometimes might also cause apparent narrowing or loss of a joint space (if the bones are now overlapping each other).

Joint space narrowing is not only caused by trauma; it is the cardinal sign of arthritis, but it may also be mimicked by poor positioning or if the X-ray beam is not centred over the joint (due to the divergence of the X-ray beam). This is the

Fig. 2.9 Cartilage (joint space); widened right glenohumeral joint space (arrows) in image **(A)** caused by a posterior dislocation, as demonstrated in the axial image **(B)**. The shape of the humeral head is also altered from normal (hopefully already seen by assessing alignment in the systematic approach). (Source: Diagnostic Imaging: Musculoskeletal Trauma, STATdx © Elsevier.)

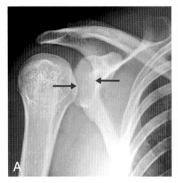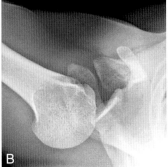

reason why when imaging a joint, dedicated images of that joint *must be taken* (e.g. a hand radiograph is not adequate for assessing the wrist). So, when joint space narrowing is identified, consider whether it may be caused by sub-optimal image quality or if there are other signs of arthritis, such as osteophytes.

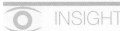

INSIGHT

Many joints, such as the acromioclavicular or distal tibiofibular joint, have a 'normal' joint width which can be considered. This is very variable and dependent on things like age, gender, and patient size, so joint measurements should be used with caution.

S – Soft Tissues (Fig. 2.10)

Whilst radiographs are not primarily used to image for soft tissue injury (ultrasound and MRI are far superior) due to a lack of radiographic contrast, the appearances of soft tissues can be a useful indicator of the underlying injury.

Following trauma, tissues bleed; bones when they fracture, and soft tissues (such as ligaments and muscles) when they are torn (sprains and strains). This bleeding can lead to the main soft tissue signs which can be assessed:

- *Soft tissue swelling* – when tissues bleed, they will swell. This can be seen clinically and radiologically at the site of injury, so its presence is a useful indicator of where the injury may have occurred.

Fig. 2.10 Soft tissues. Right knee soft tissue swelling (arrow) and enlargement and opacity of the suprapatellar bursa (*) consistent with an effusion **(A)**.
The left lateral wrist **(B)** demonstrates a lucency (hollow arrow) in the soft tissues consistent with air – indicating this is an open fracture. (Source: Diagnostic Imaging: Musculoskeletal Trauma, STATdx © Elsevier; Diagnostic Imaging: Musculoskeletal Non-Trauma, STATdx © Elsevier.)

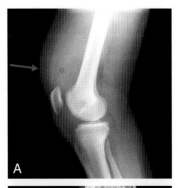

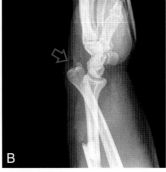

- *Displacement or obliteration of soft tissue planes* – despite soft tissues having similar densities and therefore demonstrating minimal contrast on radiographs, there is still sufficient difference to see some soft tissue planes such as between muscles and subcutaneous adipose (fatty) tissue. Displacement of these normal planes, or even their lack of visualisation, can be an indicator of underlying injury; the elevation of the fat pads in the elbow is one example (see Chapter 4).
- *Joint effusions* – caused when there is increased fluid within a joint; specifically, when this is blood, it is known as a *haemarthrosis*. Appears as an increased brightness within the joint capsule and may be associated with displacement of soft tissue planes. Common sites include the knee, elbow, and ankle. Should be considered very suspicious for underlying fracture when there is a history of trauma.

In addition, there is the potential for radiolucent air to be introduced into soft tissues in *open fractures* (Fig. 2.10). Normally these fractures will be fairly obvious, but the recognition that it is an open fracture is very significant clinically.

S – Significant Areas

Hopefully, after following the previous steps, all abnormalities on the image will have been identified. However, for each body part there are a number of well-known injuries that are very subtle, occult (invisible on imaging), or commonly missed. Similarly, there are some anatomical structures which are very significant if injured. These are known as *review areas*, and we will consider them for each individual body part in subsequent chapters.

Review the significant areas – at the end of each systematic approach, go back and check each of these review areas a second time. Make a concerted effort to inspect them.

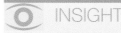

INSIGHT

In summary, when assessing radiographs of the skeletal system:
- *STOP!* Ignore any obvious abnormalities. Take a systematic approach and note anything as you go along.
- *A – adequacy*: assess the image quality and consider how it might affect interpretation. Follow a standard image quality checklist.
- *A – alignment*: check the shape of bones and alignment of joints. Are any lines/angles disrupted?
- *B – bones*: look at each bone in turn; look around the cortex of the bone for steps, lumps, or interruptions. Look inside the bones for any change in texture or disruption of the trabecular pattern.
- *C – cartilage*: assess the joint spaces; are they widened or narrowed?
- *S – soft tissues*: assess the soft tissue structures/planes. Is there any swelling, displacement, or abnormal density?
- *S – significant areas*: check the review areas, sites of significant or commonly missed injury.

In subsequent chapters we will look at specific areas to consider for each projection, but this standard approach should be the basis for the interpretation of all skeletal radiographs.

This appears a lot to consider, but by following a set approach it is far less likely that pathology will be missed, and repetition does help speed up the process over time. Any abnormalities identified can be used to make a conclusion on the image: normal or abnormal? Do we need to do anything else, such as (depending on your role):

- Identify to the referring clinician using a radiology abnormality detection system (RADS) such as a preliminary clinical evaluation (PCE)? (See Chapter 10.)
- Manage the patient?
- Flag the abnormality to a clinician?
- Take any additional projections/images?

This is the final stage of the image checklist.

Further Reading

Harcus, J. (2022). *Bones and joints: a guide for students* (8th ed). Elsevier.

FRACTURES AND JOINT TRAUMA

3

CHAPTER CONTENTS

 INSIGHT

Before understanding the mechanism of injury, an appreciation of bone structure is important. In simple terms, bone consists of cancellous and cortical bone; refer to Chapter 2, page 22 , in (cortex). Microscopically, bone is made up of Haversian (osteon) units. Appreciating the fact that normal bone has a cortical margin can assist us in determining whether a bone is fractured or not. A common error is considering accessory ossicles, sesamoid bones, and unfused apophysis to be fractures. The one thing that all these have in common is that they have a cortical margin, whereas the end of an acute fracture does not, as seen in Fig. 3.1.

Fig. 3.1 Avulsion fracture and accessory ossicle.
The red arrow represents an avulsion fracture where the end of the edges of the fracture does not have a cortical margin present. Compare this to the accessory ossicle represented by the green arrow, which has a cortical margin fully surrounding it. This is not foolproof, but it is the case in acute injuries. In cases of chronic avulsion fractures a cortical margin can develop. (Source: Fracture Management for Primary Care, Third Edition, 2018.)

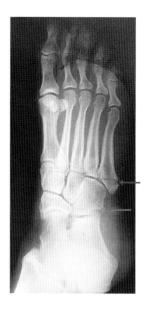

The radiolucent appearance of vascular lines can be confused with a fracture. These lines tend to run along the long axis of long bone and represent the path of nutrient vessels within bone (Fig. 2.4, Chapter 2).

Transverse radiopaque (sclerotic) lines visualised on bone can be confused for fractures. The reason for the appearance of the growth arrest lines (Harris lines, Parke Lines) is not fully understood (Fig 3.2).

Awareness of these aspects is necessary so that normal variants are not confused with bony injury.

Fig. 3.2 A and B Harris lines. Sclerotic lines can be clearly seen on the images of the tibia, indicating a period of increased bone being laid down, likely following a period of growth arrest. (Source: Skeletal Imaging: Atlas of the Spine and Extremities, Second Edition, 2011.)

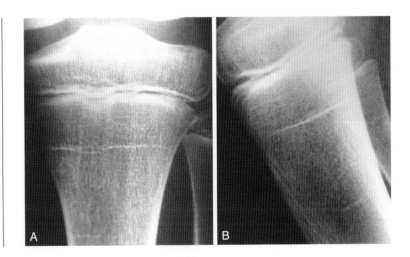

STRESS ON BONE

One factor required for healthy bone is the application of stress through forces. The ability of bone to cope with the demands placed upon it can be referred to as the integrity of bone. Failure for stress to be placed results in a loss of bone mineral density and is termed *disuse osteoporosis*; this was a problem for early astronauts and individuals who lose the use of their limbs or are immobilised for a long period of time.

Wolff's law states that bone mineral density is affected by forces (Fig. 3.3). Bones have evolved in order to cope with the forces placed on them. When bone is observed closely, the trabecular pattern is arranged in a regular way to negate the forces placed upon it.

Fig. 3.3 A–C Wolff's law demonstrated diagrammatically (A), in a specimen of bone (B) and radiographically of a specimen. These images show the arrangement of trabecular patterns in order to counteract forces placed on them. (Sources: Contemporary Orthodontics, Fourth Edition, 2007; Bullough PG: Orthopedic Pathology, Fifth Edition, St. Louis, 2010, Mosby.)

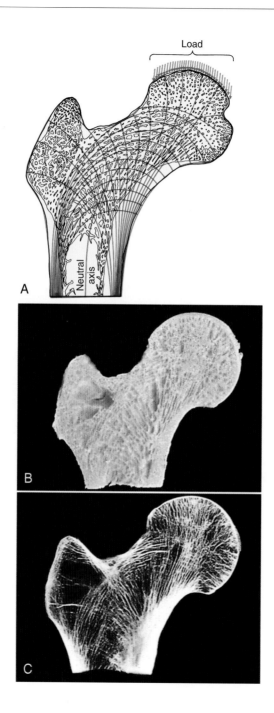

INSIGHT

Bone consists of organic and inorganic components. This ensures the integrity of the bone by providing both strength and elasticity.

There are aspects of bone that will resist compressive forces, others that resist tensile forces, and those that resist rotational forces in order for bone to maintain its integrity when encountering forces. Excessive force results in compromising the integrity of the bone and failure causing a fracture.

The type of fracture that results will be dependent on several factors:

- The intensity of the force will determine the type of fracture; a large force will result in the bone fracturing into many pieces (comminuted fracture).
- Type and direction of force, as can be seen in Fig. 3.4. The direction of force will influence the type of fracture sustained.

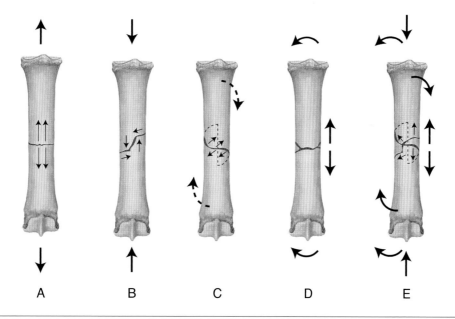

Fig. 3.4 Forces and type of resultant fracture. A represents a tension force, **B** a compressive force, **C** a torsion force, **D** a bending force, and **E** a combined force. (Source: Equine Surgery, Fifth Edition, 2019.)

Injury depends not only on the integrity of bone but also on the integrity of associated structures and is affected by the following:

- Alteration of bone. Any aspects – for example, pathology, such as osteoporosis – which alter the integrity of bone will increase the risk of fracture.

- The position of the limb at the time of impact. For example, a fall on an outstretched hand (FOOSH) can result in different bones being fractured depending on whether the initial impact was on the medial or lateral aspect of the hand.
- Structure involved. Structure associated with bones – for example, ligaments, sutures or cartilage, having less integrity than bone – could be disrupted with or without the involvement of bone.
- Shape of structure. Fig. 3.4 represents long bone, and this results in certain fracture patterns dependent on force applied. The pelvis, which is a ring structure, has the force distributed differently when compared to long bone, resulting in different fracture patterns due to loss of structural integrity.

 INSIGHT

Gravity is constantly acting on the body and therefore causing compressive forces. Gravity is acting on our bone in a downwards direction whilst our bones are resisting these forces and are hence able to withstand compressive forces to a greater extent than tensile and shear forces.

Forces can simply be divided into: tension; compressive; torsion; shear; bending; and combined, as seen in Fig. 3.4. A shear force which is not represented is a force applied at right angles to the long axis of the bone. In long bone this results in oblique spiral fracture, similar in appearance to that represented by Fig. 3.4C.

A hierarchy of bone susceptible to fracture is as follows: shearing forces are most likely to cause fractures, followed by tensile forces, and finally compression forces.

Compressive Forces

Forces that oppose one another towards the centre of a structure can be considered compressive forces. These can result in oblique fractures in long bone, open book fractures of the pelvis, and collapsed vertebrae (Fig. 3.5A, B and C).

Fig. 3.5 A–C Compressive force injury. As can be seen, the same force can result in different injury patterns. In **A,** long bone an oblique fracture is present. In **B,** the pelvis is a ring structure and results in two fractures both involving joints and results in an open book fracture. **C** is indicative of loss of structural intergrity, typical of a compression fracture. (Sources: The Elements of Fracture Fixation, Fourth Edition, 2019; Crash Course: Rheumatology and Orthopaedics, Fourth Edition, 2019; Musculoskeletal Imaging: The Core Requisites, Fifth Edition, 2022.)

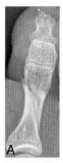

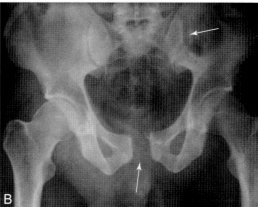

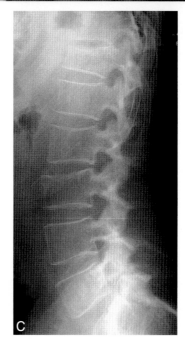

Tension Forces

This is opposite to compressive forces, where the forces that oppose one another away from centre and are trying to tear the bone part, causing a transverse fracture (Fig. 3.6A and B). This type of force causes avulsion fractures where the force from a tendon or ligament is sufficient to cause a fragment of bone to become detached from the rest of the bone (Fig. 3.1). These fractures can occur anywhere.

Fig. 3.6 A and B transverse fracture as a result of tension force. (Sources: Fracture Management: For Primary Care and Emergency Medicine, Fourth Edition, 2020; Fundamental Orthopedic Management for the Physical Therapist Assistant, Fifth Edition, 2022.)

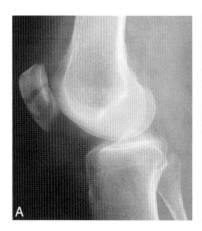
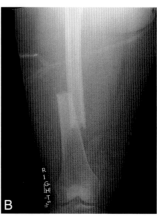

Torsion Forces

Torsion forces are twisting forces and result in a spiral fracture (Fig. 3.7).

Fig. 3.7 Spiral fracture. The twisting pattern can be noted. The varying thickness of bone results in differences in radiopacity and radiolucency, and when the two fragments are aligned, they can be mistaken for multiple fragments. (Source: Musculoskeletal Imaging: The Core Requisites, Fifth Edition, 2022.)

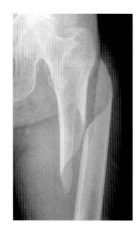

Shear Forces

Forces that act along a plane of the body or parallel to a surface are known as shear forces. Shear forces will result in spiral fractures at 45° to the long axis of the long bone.

Bending Forces

These forces result in deformity of the bone. As bone has an elastic property to it, this allows the bone to bend and absorb forces. The resulting fracture would be transverse. This is demonstrated in Fig. 3.8A, which demonstrates the direction of the impact force on the bone. Fig. 3.8B shows the bone bending to compensate for the force. The bone surface nearest to the force is placed under compression forces, whereas the surface furthest from the force is placed under tension forces. As previously described bone is less resilient to tension forces than compression forces and the bone integrity is lost at the surface experiencing tension forces Fig. 3.8C. This results in the bone surface being compromised at the point where tensile forces are present; this spreads across the bone, resulting in a transverse fracture Fig. 3.8D.

Now we will consider what happens if another force is present, as in the case of gravity (Fig. 3.9A–D). Compressional and tension forces will be present due to the direction of the impact force. In addition to this, the gravitational force will be adding compression force to the bone (Fig. 3.9A). As in the previous example, the bone will fail at the point where there is a tension force, resulting in a transverse component across the bone. Closer to the impact a combination of the forces will result in an oblique fracture in the direction of the vector of the combined forces. This results in a transverse and oblique component.

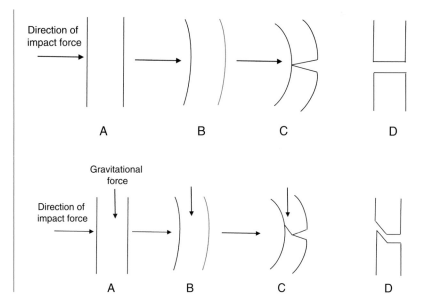

Fig. 3.8 Direction of impact force. **A, B** Red represents surface experiencing tension force. **C** Loss of bone integrity resulting in fracture. **D** Transverse fracture.

Fig. 3.9 Direction of impact force. **A, B** Red represents surface experiencing tension force. **C** Loss of bone integrity resulting in transverse fracture component. The additional compression force causes an oblique component to the fracture. **D** Transverse and oblique fracture.

INSIGHT

As we see from the above, appreciating the force of impact will help us to appreciate the pattern of the fracture appearance. In addition to this, the two example in Fig. 3.9 show when a fracture occurs in the diaphysis of the bone. Trabecular bone adds a framwork of support, and this results in the patterns not following those described. What can be appreciated from this overview is the complex nature of fractures.

The butterfly fracture is an example of the action of multiple forces, as seen in Fig. 3.10. What is of interest to note in Fig. 3.10 is the bone which is load bearing; that is, the tibia having compression forces due to gravity and shear force due to the impact results in a typical appearance of a butterfly fracture, whereas the fibula, which is non–weight-bearing in this instance, appears to have been spared.

Fig. 3.10 Butterfly fracture. (Source: Skeletal Trauma, First Edition, 2020.)

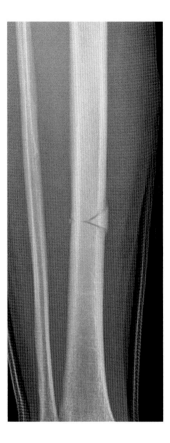

Types of fractures:

Avulsion fracture: a result of force applied to tendon being sufficient to pull a fragment of bone from its site of attachment (Fig. 3.1).

Closed: where the fracture does not result in rupturing of the skin.

Open/compound: results in rupturing of the skin, commonly by a bone fragment.

Transverse: a fracture that is perpendicular to the long axis of the bone and is from a force in the same direction (Fig. 3.6A and B).

Spiral: a fracture resulting from a rotational force twisting along the long axis of the bone (Fig. 3.7).

Comminuted: as a result of severe force causing the bone to be broken into many pieces.

Impacted: usually as a result of a force along the long axis of the bone driving one end of the bone into itself.

Greenstick: an incomplete fracture in bone of children resulting in buckling or bowing of the bone (Fig. 3.12B).

Oblique: the fracture is at an angle to the long axis of the bone (Fig. 3.5A).

Stress: a fracture as a result of repetitive forces.

Pathological: result from bone integrity being compromised due to pathology.

Osteochondral fracture: these fractures involve both bone and cartilage and will be considered later in this chapter under the Salter-Harris fractures.

 INSIGHT

A fracture can be more than one of the types described; for example, a fracture can be a closed transverse fracture.

Understanding the mechanism of injury can aid us to appreciate what to expect in terms of image appearances.

By considering forces we can begin to appreciate the appearance of fractures and what type of injury we may expect to be present. But as we have alluded, these are much more complex, as there are numerous factors to consider. In addition to this, one mechanism of injury can result in a variety of areas being a potential areas of injury as demonstrated in Fig. 3.11A & B.

As previously stated, a fracture results when bone fails to resist the force being applied. Just like any system, failure will occur at its weakest point. This is why we come across so many common sites of injury, for example, scaphoid or Colles fractures. The two examples given can be caused by the same mechanism of injury: a fall on an outstretched hand. If the force is too great for the bone to withstand, then a fracture will occur. In order to understand the reason why the same mechanism of injury results in different injuries, we not only need to appreciate forces, but we have to consider other factors. In this case one consideration is the integrity of the bone due to aging. A person who is elderly may be suffering from osteoporosis, which impacts the integrity of their bone, resulting in the weakened area being the distal radius, hence a Colles fracture. An individual whose bones have not been affected by osteoporosis and a relatively young adult may suffer a scaphoid fracture.

The force on the bones of the forearm (radius and ulna) acts in a downwards direction. The force will be transferred along the limb. The weakest point will depend on factors such as the integrity of bone. The shaft of long bone has evolved to resist compressive forces, and it is the cancellous bone which tends to fail first. If the cancellous bone has been reduced, as in the case of osteoporosis, this further reduces the integrity of the bone, creating an area of weakness.

 INSIGHT

Cancellous bone has a faster rate of turnover than cortical bone. As a result, the effects of osteoporosis will disrupt cancellous bone before cortical bone.

As can be seen from Fig. 3.11A, the overall force is in a direction towards the ground. The weakest area in this case as previously established is the cancellous bone, in this case located at the distal end of the wrist. The fixed point is at the distal end, where the hand is in contact with the ground. This results in the proximal aspect of the wrist continuing to travel in a downwards direction resulting in excessive force and the bone to fracture, the proximal end of the wrist being forced anteriorly, with the distal fragment displaced posteriorly (Fig. 3.11B), giving the classic dinner fork deformity of a Colles fracture (Fig. 3.12).

Fig. 3.11 A Diagramatic representation of fall on an outstretched hand. The arrow represents gravitational force. **B** Displacement occuring due to force.

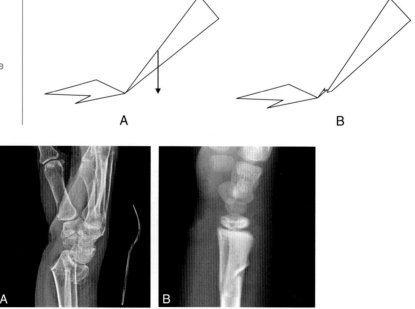

Fig. 3.12 A and B FOOSH. In **A** we note the bone appears osteopaenic, and this is of an elderly patient with typical appearances of a Colles fracture, with the distal fragment being posteriorly displaced. There are breaks in the cortical bone. The appearance is similar to the extent in **B**, which is of a paediatric patient, as noted by the presence of epiphyses. What is different in this case is that the cortex is buckled posteriorly and remains intact on the anterior aspect. (Source: Diagnostic Imaging: Musculoskeletal Trauma, Third Edition, 2021.)

Salter-Harris Fractures

Salter-Harris fractures are a group of fractures occurring in bone which has not fused at the point of an apophysis. Salter-Harris fractures can be classified into five types as demonstrated in Fig. 3.13A. SALTER can be used as a mnemonic to help identify the five types.

Type I occurs in a fracture straight across the cartilage growth plate. Can be considered a transverse fracture (S – straight across or slipped).

Type II occurs in a fracture of the bone above the growth plate and through part of the growth plate. Just as in type I, an aspect of this fracture is through the growth plate (A – above).

Type III occurs in a fracture of the bone lower than the growth plate and through part of the growth plate (L – lower).

Type IV occurs in a fracture through everything that is bone above and lower than the growth plate, as well as through the growth plate; that is, it involves the diaphysis, metaphysis, and epiphysis (TE – Through Everything).

Type V causes compression (ramming) of the diaphysis and epiphysis into the growth plate (metaphysis), that is, compressing the metaphysis (rammed – R).

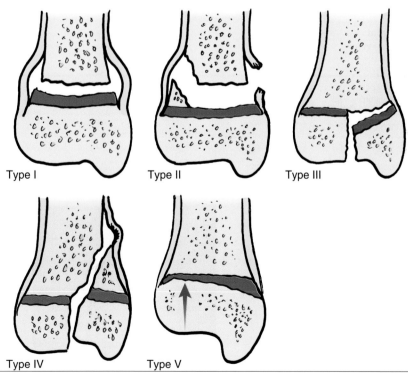

Type I Type II Type III

Type IV Type V

Fig. 3.13 Salter-Harris fracture classification. (Source: Fundamental Orthopedic Management for the Physical Therapist Assistant, Fifth Edition.)

Type I	Type II	Type III	Type IV	Type V
S	A	L	TE	R
Straight across, slipped	Above (growth plate)	Lower (than growth plate)	Through everything	Rammed

When growth plates are present, fractures can be difficult to appreciate due to the inability to visualise cartilage on radiographic images. Around the growth plate there are cortical margins which aid in distinguishing between the two.

INSIGHT

It is important to appreciate that in children and adolescents the bone model is present but in a cartilage form. As cartilage is not visible on a radiographic image, any fracture of the cartillage will also not be visible.

Soft Tissue Signs of Fractures

We need to remember that bone is living tissue. As such, any injury to bone, in this case fracture, will result in disruption to blood vessels. The disruption to the blood vessels will result in immediate swelling. In cases where the fractured bone is across an articular surface, the bleeding increases the volume inside the joint capsule, as in some elbow fractures resulting in raised fat pads Fig. 3.14A–C. This would be an intra-articular fracture. Alternatively fractures can be

Fig. 3.14 A–C Elbow fat pads. Diagram **A** represents the normal location of the fat pads. Diagram **B** demonstrates raised fat pads due to effusion within the joint capsule. Image **C** shows the appearance of raised fat pads due to the radiolucent appearance of fat. This is an indication of the presence of an injury. (Source: Tachdjian's Pediatric Orthopaedics: From the Texas Scottish Rite Hospital for Children, Sixth Edition, 2022.)

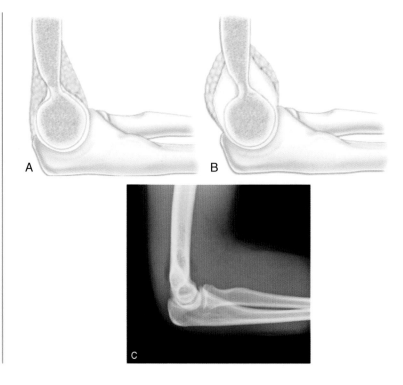

Fig. 3.15 A and B Ankle injury. In **A** note the soft tissue swelling around the lateral maleolus. Normally the soft tissue is in close proximity to the lateral malleolus. Upon closer inspection a radiolucent line can be noted, as well as minimal cortical displacement. **B** further confirms the injury with the visualisation of a step in the cortex on the posterior aspect of the fibula. (Source: Skeletal Trauma, First Edition, 2020.)

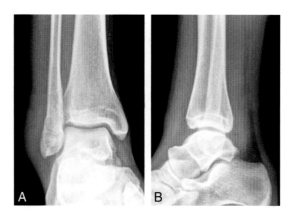

extra-articular. As has been established, forces are involved in fractures; these forces will disrupt not only bone but also the surrounding tissue. The disruption of surrounding tissue will also contribute to swelling as seen in Fig 3.15.

 INSIGHT

Not all fractures are visible. Reasons why fractures may not be visible include: the sensitivity of X-ray imaging; and fractures involving structures that are not visualised on X-ray images; for example, cartilage is difficult to detect. If there is no displacement of bone, then other factors are relied on, for example, soft tissue signs to indicate the presence of injury.

In cases where fractures are suspected and not visualised, a follow-up examination may be required at a later date to assess if there is any further evidence of fracture, for example, visualisation of fracture through the fracture healing process, in terms of callus formation (Fig. 3.16A and B).

Double Lines

As we have seen earlier, fractures can present in different ways depending upon the force applied. If you are unaware of what has occurred, it can be quite easy to misinterpret a single fracture as two fractures. A single fracture can present as a double line on an image if the X-ray beam does not travel straight through the fracture but at an angle. This occurs due to the aspect of the fracture closest to the X-ray beam being in a different place to the aspect furthest from the X-ray beam.

Fig. 3.16 A & B. A demonstrates an extremely faint transverse line on the diaphysis of the second metatarsal demonstrating a fracture. **B** is a follow-up radiographic image where callus formation has started. Note the difference in the cortical margin of the second metatarsal compared to other similar metatarsals, thus confirming the original presence of the injury. (Source: Musculoskeletal Imaging, Second Edition, 2015.)

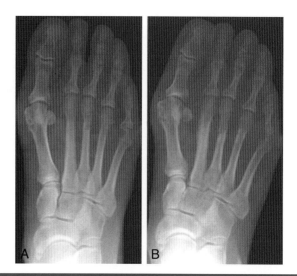

 INSIGHT

We need to appreciate that X-ray images are two-dimensional representations of three-dimensional structures. As such, the projection and beam orientation will impact image appearance.

This is why it is essential to view all projections and assimilate the information in order to reach the correct conclusion (Fig. 3.17A & B), and why in most instances we take two images that are orthogonal to one another.

Fig. 3.17 A & B. The importance of two views. As can be seen from the two views, reviewing the **A** anteroposterior projection of the tibia and fibula, the image could be considered being normal. There does not appear to be any apparent disruption to the cortical margins of the bone. On the **B** lateral image a totally different conclusion is reached, as there is clear evidence of a radiolucent line in the tibia demonstrating a spiral fracture. To reinforce the point in Chapter 1, page 9, collect all the evidence before making your conclusion. (Source: Diagnostic Imaging: Musculoskeletal, STATdx © Elsevier.)

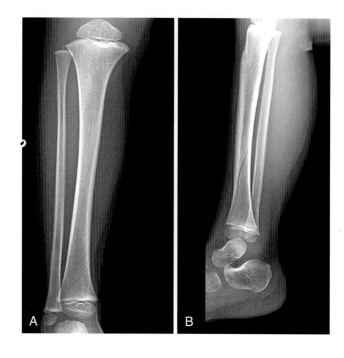

CONCLUSION

As can be seen throughout this chapter, there are many aspects that need to be understood in order to appreciate how injuries are presented on radiographic images. Even when there does not appear to be any bony evidence of injury, it is important to critically review the whole image for signs that may indicate that there is an injury present. Remember, not all fractures are always visible on radiographic images or a single view.

UPPER LIMB

4

In this chapter we will consider the interpretation of skeletal radiographs of the upper limb (note that the shoulder joint and bones of the shoulder girdle are considered separately in Chapter 5). The upper limb is extremely prone to injury due to its extrinsic position and forces placed upon it, particularly in falls.

 INSIGHT

Different patterns of injury following a similar mechanism of injury typically differ according to a patient's age. In the upper limb this is particularly evident following a 'FOOSH' (*fall onto outstretched hand*) injury. Most commonly, the following types of injury usually occur at the approximate ages:

- **3–8 years** – Torus/buckle fracture distal radius
- **5–7 years** – Supracondylar (elbow) fracture
- **8–16 years** – Salter-Harris 2 fracture of the distal radius
- **17–30 years** – Scaphoid fracture (or radial head fracture)
- **30–40 years** – Radial head fracture
- **40–70 years** – Colles (distal radius) fracture
- **>70 years** – Neck of humerus fracture

As with a number of these concepts, however, this is certainly not a hard-and-fast rule. There are numerous other potential injuries which can occur, and injuries can occur at different ages, but it is a start!

HUMERUS

The humerus is the largest bone of the upper limb. As a large long bone, fractures are commonly obvious, and a typical systematic approach should identify them; however, you should be mindful to review the entire image.

Systematic Approach

Radiographic appearances of the humerus (Fig. 4.1).

Anteroposterior and lateral projections

Follow the standard approach to the AABCSS in addition to:

Adequacy	• Are both the elbow and glenohumeral joint included on the image? • Are the proximal humerus and elbow joint grossly AP/lateral dependent on the projection? • Is the humerus clear from the ribs?
Alignment	• Are the glenohumeral and elbow joints grossly aligned (remember, these are not dedicated projections)? • Is the radial head articulating with the capitulum (on both projections) – radiocapitellar line (see page 50)? • Is there any rotation between the glenohumeral and elbow joint (i.e. are they both grossly AP/lateral)?
Bones	• Assess the humerus • Assess the visible scapula, clavicle, ribs, and forearm
Cartilage (Joint spaces)	• Not dedicated views, difficult to assess joint spaces
Soft tissues	• Is there soft tissue swelling, particularly over the proximal and mid humerus? • Are the soft tissue planes displaced?
Significant areas	• Look for evidence of rib fractures • The proximal humerus, particularly the greater tuberosity • Is there any pathology in the visible lung (e.g. pneumothorax)? • Do we need dedicated shoulder/elbow projections?

Fig. 4.1 AP and lateral humerus projections: systematic approach.
Alignment – glenohumeral and elbow joints aligned? Radiocapitellar line (dotted line). Bones – carefully check **ALL** of the visible bones. Cartilage – any gross narrowing/widening of the glenohumeral and elbow joint spaces? Soft tissues – is there any soft tissue swelling? Significant areas – ribs, lung, proximal humerus/greater tuberosity (arrow), do we need dedicated shoulder/elbow projections? (Source: Bontrager's Handbook of Radiographic Positioning and Techniques, Tenth Edition, 2021.)

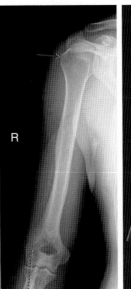
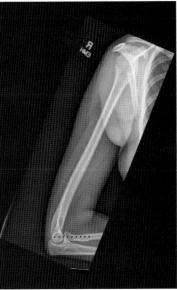

Fractures

As a strong bone, fractures typically only occur due to high-velocity/high-energy forces or where the bone is weakened due to underlying pathology (e.g. osteoporosis) or age.

Fractures typically occur either of the shaft (diaphysis) and will be fairly obvious, or proximally (neck of humerus), or distally. The latter two will be considered when looking at the elbow and shoulder (Chapter 5), respectively, since dedicated projections should be used to assess them.

Shaft/Diaphysis Fracture (Fig. 4.2)

Typical mechanism of injury:
- High energy; for example, road traffic collisions
- Low energy, such as falls, due to osteoporosis or advanced age
- Pathological due to underlying pathology

Clinical presentation:
- Pain, swelling, and foreshortening of arm
- Neuropathy if injury to radial nerve

Appearance:
- Midshaft (75% in middle third); distal to the surgical neck and proximal to the supracondylar ridge
- Transverse most commonly; may be oblique or spiral
- Usually obvious due to marked displacement caused by deltoid, biceps brachii, and brachialis muscles

Fig. 4.2 Right humeral shaft fracture; AP (A) and lateral (B) projections. This oblique fracture demonstrates classic medial and proximal displacement due to muscular contractions. Note that the exclusion of the glenohumeral joint and humeral head means assessment of rotation at the fracture cannot be assessed radiographically. It is clear why these types of fractures are often associated with neurovascular injury. (Source: From STATdx © Elsevier.)

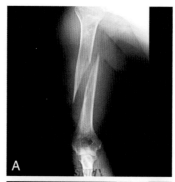

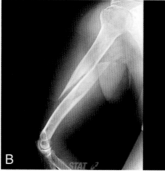

- Typically varus angulation (elbow deviated towards midline) with medial and proximal displacement of the distal fracture fragment, again due to muscle contraction

 INSIGHT

As with a lot of large long bone fractures, associated neurovascular injury must be considered due to the close relationship of the humerus and radial nerve and brachial artery (Fig. 4.3).

Fig. 4.3 Posterior view of the left humerus. Note the close relation of the radial nerve and brachial artery, which may be injured with humeral shaft fractures. (Source: From STATdx © Elsevier)

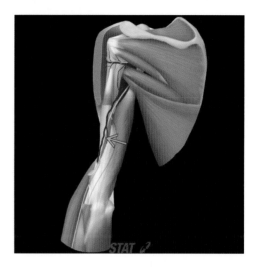

ELBOW

The elbow joint is a complex structure which, like many large joints in general, makes image interpretation potentially challenging. The elbow is comprised of two separate joints: the articulation between the humerus, radius, and ulna (synovial hinge); and the proximal radio-ulna joint (synovial pivot). Differences between paediatric and adult anatomy add a further level of complexity, and we will consider specific aspects of the paediatric elbow separately.

Adequacy

Whilst image quality is important for all radiographic examinations, for joints like the elbow, positioning in particular can make a huge difference in the ability to confidently identify or rule out injury. Patient presentation and pain can make positioning difficult, so it is important to consider the effect image quality has.

INSIGHT

It is important to systematically review all images produced, even if they are not optimal and need to be repeated. Subtle fractures such as those of the radial head might potentially be visible on sub-optimal images even if there are not on more adequate projections. Alternatively an additional projection might help exclude a suspected injury seen on another projection. Use all information available to you.

Some specific points to consider when assessing adequacy of the elbow.

Anteroposterior projection:

- ensure the forearm is supinated so that the radial head and neck are clearly visible; there will normally be a degree of overlap with the proximal ulna
- extension of the elbow allows visualisation of the joint space and articular surfaces

Lateral projection:

- a 'true' lateral is very important for identifying minimally displaced distal humerus fractures in particular; look for superimposition of the capitulum and trochlea and the classic '*figure of 8*' appearance (Fig. 4.6)
- appropriate exposure and image processing ensures soft tissue structures, which can aid in interpretation, are visible

Alignment

As well as assessing the normal alignment of the elbow joint and articulation between the capitulum and radial head, the trochlea and proximal ulna, and the proximal ulna and radial head, there are some particular lines which are useful in image interpretation.

Radiocapitellar line (Figs. 4.4 and 4.5):

- the articular surfaces of the radial head and capitulum should *always* be congruent. Lack of congruity suggests radial head dislocation and may be associated with other fractures in the forearm (and may warrant additional dedicated images)
- *a line drawn through the long axis of the radial neck should always bisect the middle of the capitulum*
- it is possible to assess this line *regardless of the projection*, so it should be assessed on projections of the humerus, elbow, and forearm – even if they are sub-optimal

Carrying angle (Fig. 4.4):

- normal valgus angle between the long axes of the humerus and ulna at the elbow joint (forearm angled more lateral than humerus)
- greater in women than men (due to width of pelvis), the average angle being 163°
- visible on anteroposterior projection; not to be confused with subluxation

Anterior humeral line (Fig. 4.5):

- *only reliable on a true lateral elbow projection*; sub-optimal positioning or non-dedicated projections render this line otherwise unreliable

Fig. 4.4 AP Elbow projection: alignment.
A, Radiocapitellar line (dotted line). A line drawn through the long axis of the radial neck bisects the middle of the capitulum.
B, Carrying angle (curved line). Normal valgus angle between long axes humerus and ulna (solid line). (Source: Bontrager's Textbook of Radiographic Positioning and Related Anatomy, Tenth Edition, 2021.)

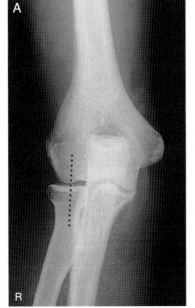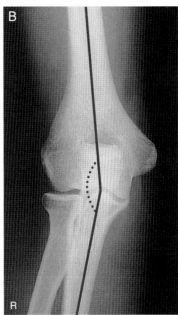

Fig. 4.5 Lateral elbow projection: alignment.
A, Radiocapitellar line (dotted line). A line drawn through the long axis of the radial neck bisects the middle of the capitulum.
B, Anterior humeral line. A line drawn down the anterior cortex of the humerus (dotted line) should bisect between the anterior and middle one-third of the capitulum (circle). (Source: Bontrager's Textbook of Radiographic Positioning and Related Anatomy, Tenth Edition, 2021.)

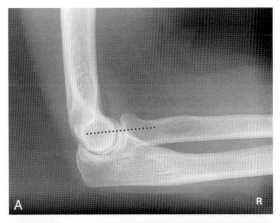

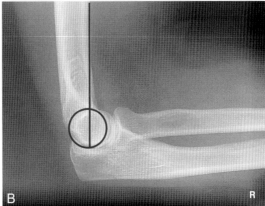

- *a line drawn along the anterior cortex of the distal humerus should normally bisect between the anterior and middle third of the capitulum* (i.e. one-third will be anterior to the line and two-thirds posterior to it)
- indicative of fracture of the distal humerus if less or more (less common) of the capitulum is seen anterior to this line

Bones

The bone's external cortex and internal texture should be carefully assessed by looking at the humerus, radius, and ulna separately. When looking at the differences between the adult and paediatric skeleton, there are marked differences in appearance, and we will consider these differences later in the chapter.

Whilst fractures of the bones around the elbow may be very obvious, there are some specific areas where more subtle (or sometimes occult) minimally displaced fractures may be demonstrated, particularly:

- The radial head and neck
- The coronoid process
- The distal humerus; particularly the anterior cortex

It is important these areas in particular are carefully scrutinised, looking for subtle fracture lines.

 INSIGHT

A pitfall when assessing the bones on the anteroposterior projection is mistaking the lucency formed by the olecranon fossa as a pathological lesion (Fig. 4.8).
Similarly, the radial tuberosity can also cause a similar appearance on the lateral (Fig. 4.9).

Cartilage

Adequate positioning of the anteroposterior and lateral projections will ensure the joint spaces between the humerus, radial head, and proximal ulna are demonstrated.

It is important to look carefully within the joint spaces to identify any small avulsion fractures/osteochondral fracture fragments which lie within the joint.

Soft Tissues

Aside from general or localised soft tissue swelling, which might indicate underlying injury, there is a specific sign which can be assessed, which, with a history of trauma, should be considered very suspicious for underlying bone or soft tissue injury.

The 'Sail Sign' (Figs. 4.6 and 4.7):

- Two articular fat pads are found within the capsule of the elbow joint; the anterior one lies within the shallow coronoid fossa of the distal humerus and the posterior fat pad within the larger olecranon fossa. They act to cushion the bones on flexion and extension of the elbow joint.

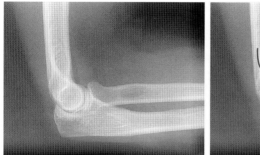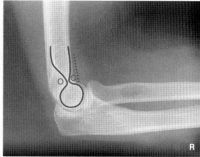

Fig. 4.6 Lateral elbow projection: soft tissues. Normal appearance of the elbow fat pads. The anterior fat pad lies within the shallower coronoid fossa (C) and is visible as a faint lucent stripe (dotted line) compared to the muscle against the humerus. The posterior fat pad lies within the deeper olecranon fossa (O) and is not normally visible. Note the normal *'figure of 8'* appearance of the distal humerus on this well-positioned lateral (solid line on B). (Source: Bontrager's Textbook of Radiographic Positioning and Related Anatomy, Tenth Edition,2021.)

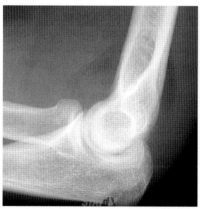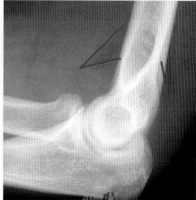

Fig. 4.7 The 'sail sign' – lateral elbow projection. There is elevation of the anterior fat pad and the posterior one is visible too, causing the classic sail sign indicating a joint effusion. With a history of trauma, this is suspicious for fracture, though in this case it is not visible. (Source: STATdx © Elsevier.)

- On a lateral elbow projection, the anterior fat pad is commonly seen as a radiolucent stripe along, and in contact with, the anterior humerus. The posterior fat pad is normally not visible, as it lies in the deeper olecranon fossa.
- An increase in joint fluid (effusion) within the joint causes these fat pads to become elevated and move out of their fossae.
- The anterior fat pad becomes elevated away from the humerus and the posterior fat pad becomes visible as another radiolucent line posterior to the distal humerus; this appearance gives rise to the *'sail sign'*.
- With a positive history of acute trauma, the *effusion* (fluid) is more likely to be blood and is known as a *haemarthrosis* and is suspicious of fracture.
- When demonstrated in the absence of a visible fracture, a possible occult radial head or supracondylar fracture should be suspected and further imaging or investigation may be required.

Whilst useful, the sail sign should be interpreted with caution for a number of reasons:

- The sign is not only caused by a fracture:
  - There may be soft tissue injury causing the bleeding not visible on radiographs.
  - The effusion (fluid) might not be blood but other types of fluid such as an excess in synovial fluid (due to arthritis) or pus (in septic arthritis); clinical history is key.
  - In significant joint injuries (e.g. dislocation) where the joint capsule is ruptured, any fluid will escape and not cause the fat pads to be elevated.
  - Injuries external to the joint capsule will not cause bleeding within the joint and therefore will not cause the sail sign.

 INSIGHT

A positive sail (fat pad) sign with a history of trauma should be considered highly suspicious for underlying bony injury, particularly of radial head or distal humerus fractures. However, a positive sail sign is not always caused by fracture and might not be evident in all injuries to the elbow joint.

Significant Areas

There are some subtle fractures that occur related to the elbow joint that should be carefully looked for. Hopefully the assessment already described will identify this but specifically assess:

- the radial head and neck for subtle steps or lucencies which may indicate a fracture
- the coronoid process; this may be avulsed and can be very difficult to identify
- the anterior cortex of the distal humerus for subtle gaps in the cortex caused by a minimally displaced distal humerus (supracondylar) fracture, particularly in paediatric patients

Systematic Approach

Radiographic appearances of the elbow joint (Figs. 4.8 and 4.9).

Anteroposterior and lateral projections

Follow the standard approach to the AABCSS in addition to:

Adequacy	• True lateral elbow projection; are the capitulum and trochlea superimposed? • Is the radial head clear from the proximal ulna (allowing for some overlap)? • Are joint spaces clear?
Alignment	• Radiocapitellar line (both projections) • Anterior humeral line (true lateral projection) • Carrying angle (anteroposterior projection)
Bones	• Assess the humerus, radius, and ulna in turn • Pay particular attention to the radial head/neck, coronoid process, articular surfaces, and anterior surface of the distal humerus • CRITOL (paediatrics only) – does the order of the ossification centres follow the typical pattern?

Cartilage (Joint spaces)	• Assess for presence of intra-articular bone fragments
Soft tissues	• Soft tissue swelling • Sail sign (lateral projection) – is there a joint effusion?
Significant areas	• Radial head and neck • Coronoid process • Anterior cortex of distal humerus

Fig. 4.8 AP elbow projection: systematic approach. Alignment – radiocapitellar line, carrying angle. Bones – humerus, radius, ulna; radial head and neck (solid line). Cartilage – any intra-articular bone fragments? Soft tissues – is there any soft tissue swelling? Significant areas – Radial head and neck, coronoid process (arrow). Note the lucency formed by the olecranon fossa (*), which may be mistaken as pathological. (Source: Bontrager's Textbook of Radiographic Positioning and Related Anatomy, Tenth Edition, 2021.)

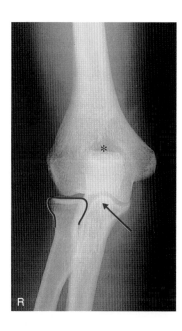

Fig. 4.9 Lateral elbow projection: systematic approach. Alignment – radiocapitellar line, anterior humeral line. Bones – humerus, radius, ulna; radial head and neck. Cartilage – any intra-articular bone fragments? Soft tissues – is there any soft tissue swelling? Joint effusion? – look for sail sign. Significant areas – radial head and neck; coronoid process (solid line); anterior cortex of distal humerus (arrow). Note the lucency formed by the radial tuberosity (*), which may be mistaken as pathological. (Source: Bontrager's Textbook of Radiographic Positioning and Related Anatomy, Tenth Edition, 2021.)

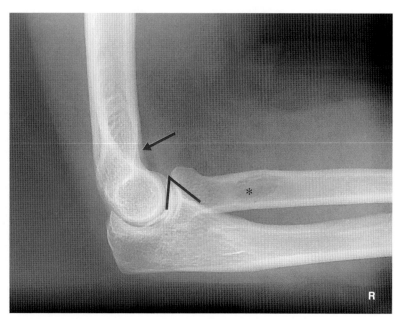

THE PAEDIATRIC ELBOW (FIG. 4.10)

Whilst all of the previous approach is relevant to both adult and paediatric elbows, there is a significant additional consideration that must be made when assessing paediatric elbow radiographs: the secondary ossification centres.

INSIGHT

It is vitally important to understand the development and radiographic appearances of bone when interpreting radiographs.

Fig. 4.10 Elbow ossification centres.
The mnemonic CRITOL is a useful tool to remember the typical order in which they appear. AP and lateral projections in a 6-year-old **(A)** and 12-year-old **(B).** Both are normal.
C – capitulum (appears age 1); *R* – radial head (age 4–5); *I* – medial (internal) epicondyle (age 4–6); *T* – trochlea (age 9–10); *O* – olecranon (9–11 years); *L* – lateral epicondyle (12 years). (Source: STATdx © Elsevier.)

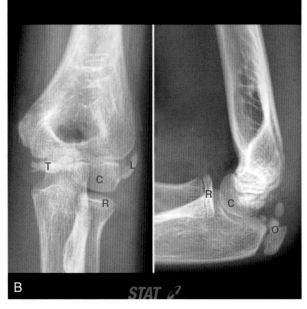

At birth, the distal end of the humerus and proximal ends of the radius and ulna are still formed by the hyaline cartilage model and have not ossified to bone. Though the cartilage structure is present, radiographically they are not evident until they have ossified.

This secondary ossification occurs at different ages and typically (though not always) follows a set pattern, commonly remembered by the mnemonic CRITOL:

C – Capitulum (ossification age 1)
R – Radial head (ossification age 4–5)
I – Internal (medial) epicondyle (ossification age 4–6)
T – Trochlea (ossification age 9–10)
O – Olecranon (ossification 9–11 years)
L – Lateral epicondyle (ossification 12 years)

- CRITOL lists the order in which the secondary ossification centres typically appear radiographically
- It can sometimes be used to identify fractures, particularly avulsion fractures, to the distal humerus
- Since they commonly appear in this order, if any bone fragments related to one of these areas are missing or appear out of sequence, then they should be considered suspicious for bone injury
- Quite often there will be localised soft tissue swelling over these types of injury, which can also be of use

As with a lot of these radiographic signs and tips, there are pitfalls that must be considered:

- CRITOL only lists the most typical order; there is overlap between ages, and it is not uncommon for there to be variations in this.
- It does not list the order in which these ossification centres fuse with the adjacent bone.
- Ossification centres might be fragmented, meaning there is more than one visible bone fragment at each site.

In summary, CRITOL is a useful tool in assessing the paediatric elbow but requires a good understanding of developmental anatomy and should be used alongside a full systematic approach.

 INSIGHT

Remember the differences in radiographic appearance between ossification centre/accessory bone and fracture; ossification centres typically appear smooth and rounded, with a cortical margin all around them, and will not fit directly onto the adjacent bone.

Fractures/Trauma

Radial Head/Neck Fracture (Fig. 4.11)   Common injury, particularly in young adults following a fall onto outstretched hand (FOOSH). Constitutes up to 50% of adult elbow fractures. Head more common in adults, neck more common in paediatric patients.

Fig. 4.11 Radial head fracture. AP projection **(A)** demonstrates a subtle lucency in the articular surface of the radial head (arrow). The lateral projection **(B)** demonstrates a positive sail sign (hollow arrows), though the fracture is not visible. These are classic appearances for a subtle radial head fracture. (Source: STATdx © Elsevier.)

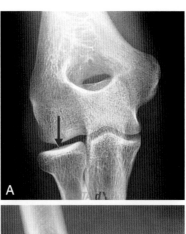

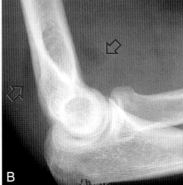

Typical mechanism of injury:
- Fall onto outstretched hand (FOOSH) – axial compression of radial head on capitulum

Clinical presentation:
- Adults and paediatrics
- Elbow pain, tenderness over radial head

Appearance:
- Often subtle and minimally displaced (may be occult on radiographs)
- May be of articular surface of head and appear as a lucent line through the cortex, or as a step in the cortex of the neck
- A positive sail sign (due to haemarthrosis) is commonly seen alongside fracture. A positive sail sign with a history of trauma and in the absence of a visible fracture should warrant further imaging/management.

Supracondylar Fracture (Figs. 4.12 and 4.13)

As the name suggests, it occurs superior to the condyles of the distal humerus, usually at the junction of the diaphysis (shaft) and metaphysis at the level of the coronoid/olecranon fossae, as this area is weaker. Severity ranges from undisplaced to significant displacement. Anterior humeral line very helpful in subtle injuries.

Fig. 4.12 Displaced supracondylar fracture; AP (A) and lateral (B) projections left elbow. There is marked medial (arrow) and posterior (hollow arrow) displacement at the site of the transverse fracture in this 5-year-old. (Source: STATdx © Elsevier.)

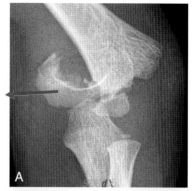

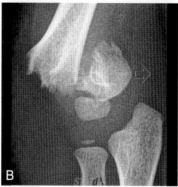

Fig. 4.13 Minimally displaced supracondylar fracture. The lateral projection in this 7-year-old demonstrates: subtle cortical irregularity of the anterior cortex (arrow); positive sail sign (hollow arrows); the anterior humeral line (dotted line) no longer bisects the capitulum (C) due to posterior displacement. There is also generalised soft tissue swelling. (Source: STATdx © Elsevier.)

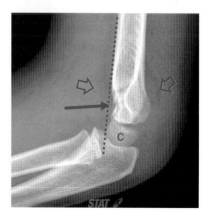

Similar mechanism of injury to radial head fracture (FOOSH) but found typically in paediatrics age 5–7 (rare in adults). Constitutes more than 50% of paediatric elbow fractures. As with other humeral fractures, there is a risk of neurovascular particularly in displaced fractures.

Typical mechanism of injury:

- FOOSH

Clinical presentation:
- Typically young children (5–7 years)
- Pain, swelling, and loss of function
- Neuropathy or discoloured/cold wrist suggestive of neurovascular injury

Appearance:
- Transverse fracture of the distal humerus with posterior displacement
- Imaging findings dependent on severity of displacement
  - Mild; disruption of anterior cortex, loss of anterior humeral line
  - Severe; obvious fracture line with posterior displacement of capitulum
  - Positive sail sign where haemarthrosis is present

Elbow Dislocation

(Fig. 4.14)

Either of the main elbow joint (articulation between the distal humerus and radius/ulna) or of the proximal radio-ulnar joint (see forearm fractures; page 70).

Up to 50% associated with bony fracture, in particular medial condyle of humerus, coronoid process, and radial head.

Typical mechanism of injury:
- Fall onto outstretched hand (FOOSH) with elbow in extension

Fig. 4.14 Elbow dislocation; right elbow. The AP **(A)** demonstrates a clear lateral dislocation of the radius and ulna in relation to the humerus. It is less obvious on the lateral **(B),** but there is an apparent widening of the joint space and loss of the radiocapitellar line on both projections (dotted line). A fracture fragment is present (arrow) though there is no donor site demonstrated. Note the lack of joint effusion (sail sign), which is not uncommon in significant injury. (Source: STATdx © Elsevier.)

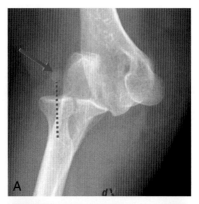

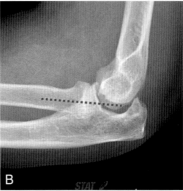

Clinical presentation:
- Young adults and paediatrics (most common dislocation in paediatrics)
- Pain, swelling, and gross deformity

Appearance:
- Loss of alignment of articular surfaces of radial head and capitellum (loss of radiocapitellar line) and olecranon of ulna and trochlea of humerus
- Usually dislocate posteriorly or posterolaterally
- Need to assess for associated bony fracture and intra-articular fragments

Olecranon Process Fracture (Figs. 4.15 and 4.16)

Typical mechanism of injury:
- Direct blow (e.g. fall onto flexed elbow)
- Forced flexion; avulsion injury caused by insertion of triceps muscles

Clinical presentation:
- More common in adults than in paediatrics
- Pain and swelling over olecranon process
- Reduced extension of elbow

Appearance:
- Transverse fracture through olecranon process; intra-articular

Fig. 4.15 Olecranon fracture. The fracture often extends into the elbow joint. Note the insertion of the tendons of the triceps muscles on the olecranon process (arrow), which can cause significant displacement of the fracture. (Source: STATdx © Elsevier.)

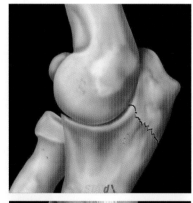

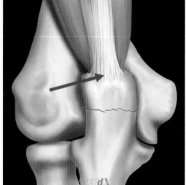

Fig. 4.16 Comminuted olecranon fracture, caused by a fall from height with multiple fragments demonstrated of the fracture. There is also a fracture of the radial neck (arrow) indicating the need for a thorough satisfaction of search. Also note the presence of a haemarthrosis (positive sail sign; hollow arrows). (Source: STATdx © Elsevier.)

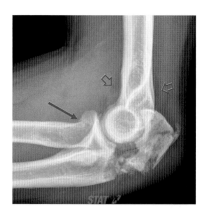

- If complete, fragment usually displaced proximally/superiorly due to traction of biceps muscle
- More obvious on lateral projection
- In paediatrics it is important not to confuse normal ossification centre with fracture (Fig. 4.10)

Condyle Fractures

(Figs. 4.17 and 4.18)

May occur of the medial or lateral condyle of the distal humerus. Though they can occur in adults, they are more common in paediatrics. Lateral condyle is more commonly affected than medial.

Fig. 4.17 Medial epicondyle fracture. It is possible to see on **(A)** how small the bony fragment is in comparison to the cartilage (shown in blue). **(B)** demonstrates a large medial condyle fracture (arrow) in a 9-year-old; the fragment has rotated from its normal orientation. Note the localised soft tissue swelling (hollow arrow). (Source: STATdx © Elsevier.)

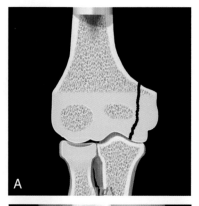

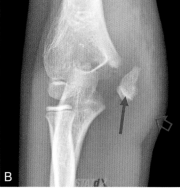

Fig. 4.18 Lateral condyle fractures; two examples.
(A) shows a subtle linear fracture fragment (arrow) adjacent to the lateral condyle in this 2-year-old. This is a fairly typical appearance in fractures in young paediatrics and may be easily missed.
(B) demonstrates a more obvious fracture of the lateral condyle (hollow arrow), which still articulates with the capitulum (C) ossification centre in a 4-year-old. The radiocapitellar line (dotted line) is disrupted. (Source: STATdx © Elsevier.)

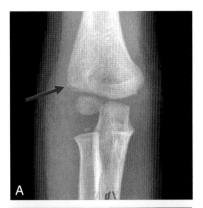

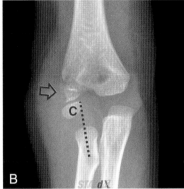

When they occur in an immature skeleton, it is important to remember that the fracture might be within the unossified hyaline cartilage (Fig. 4.17) and therefore not directly visible on radiographs; they are classified as Salter-Harris fractures, since they involve the physeal plate of the ossification centre.

In paediatrics they can lead to growth disturbances if not diagnosed and treated appropriately.

Typical mechanism of injury:
- Lateral condyle; direct blow to lateral forearm causing traction of lateral elbow; FOOSH
- Medial condyle; direct blow to medial forearm; FOOSH

Clinical presentation:
- Most commonly age 4–10 years (lateral) and 7–14 years (medial)
- Localised pain and swelling

Appearance:
- Best demonstrated on AP usually
- Dependent on size and location of fracture; ranges from very small to large bone fragments, or there is no visible fracture if only cartilage is involved
- May demonstrate as a small linear fracture fragment adjacent to the respective condyle

- If there is a cartilage fracture only, then the ossification centre (if visible) will be displaced from its normal position, or even missing (use CRITOL to help decide whether it should be present).
- Localised soft tissue swelling and positive sail sign are common.

 INSIGHT

Fractures involving cartilage can be underestimated on radiographs. Whilst the bony fracture fragment might appear very small, the cartilage involvement (which is not visible) may be very large. It might be likened to an iceberg; the bit we can see is only the tip of it!

Medial Epicondyle Avulsion Fracture

(Fig. 4.19)

Involves the medial epicondyle ossification centre of the distal humerus; the fracture is of the unossified hyaline cartilage and therefore not directly visible on radiographs.

Can be traumatic and acute, or chronic due to repetitive stress. Can lead to growth disturbances if not diagnosed and treated appropriately.

Typical mechanism of injury:
- acute – FOOSH with elbow flexed or throwing injury
- chronic – repetitive overarm throwing (sometimes called Little-Leaguer elbow due to association with young baseball players)

Clinical presentation:
- Most commonly age 8–14
- Localised pain and swelling

Appearance:
- Best demonstrated on AP usually
- Displacement of normal medial epicondyle ossification centre. Normally, according to CRITOL, the medial epicondyle should be present if the trochlea is
- May be further away from medial condyle than normal or completely displaced (even in the joint space)
- Localised soft tissue swelling and positive sail sign common

Fig. 4.19 Medial epicondyle avulsion.
The medial epicondyle (arrow) is displaced from its normal position adjacent to the medial condyle (MC), compared the appearances of Fig. 4.10. Note the focal soft tissue swelling medially too. (Source: STATdx © Elsevier.)

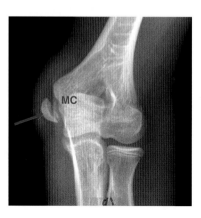

FOREARM

The forearm should be considered a fibro-osseous (i.e. made of bone and fibrous/soft tissue) structure comprised of the radius and ulna bones which are connected distally by the distal radioulnar joint (DRUJ) at the wrist and proximally by the proximal radioulnar joint. As such, a systematic approach is essential; if one injury is identified, look for more.

Adequacy

It is important to ensure that both elbow and wrist joints are included on the images. Although not dedicated projections of either, and it is difficult to get true AP and lateral images of both at the same time, injuries to these areas can still often be identified. The projections should demonstrate both the bones and joints at 90° to each other, and the forearm should be supinated on the antero-posterior projection so that the radius and ulna are not overlapping/crossing.

Alignment

The radius and ulna typically have a slight varus angulation in them, but look for any excessive deviation of the bone's shape, especially in paediatrics where plastic bowing (see fractures, page 69) may occur.

Though it is difficult to achieve a true AP/lateral of both joints on the relevant projection, assess for gross rotation between the elbow and wrist.

It is also important to assess the radiocapitellar line (see page 50) as dislocations of the radial head may be identified despite forearm views not being dedicated to imaging the elbow. This can be assessed on both the AP and lateral projections and should always apply regardless of position.

Similarly, despite not being a dedicated projection of the wrist, it is important to assess the alignment of the distal radius and ulna with each other and the carpals. In particular, the distal radial and ulna should be superimposed on the lateral projection (take into account the positioning), and on the anteroposterior, the radial angle (see page 73) should intersect the head of ulna. Failure to do so may indicate dislocation of the DRUJ.

Bones

Most fractures tend to occur in the middle or distal third of the bones, though they can occur anywhere, so it is important to carefully review all aspects. Pay particular attention to common areas of fracture such as the radial head at the elbow and both styloid processes at the wrist.

Typically fractures of long bones like the radius and ulna are quite obvious, but minimally displaced fractures which commonly may be seen in paediatrics may not be complete or cause large amounts of displacement and so may be harder to visualise. Such fractures often appear only as 'bumps' in the cortex.

Remember to assess all visible bones in turn, including those at the edges of the image.

Cartilage

As these are not dedicated projections of the elbow/wrist joint, subtle (or even gross) joint abnormalities may not be evident. However, it is still important to assess the visible joint spaces for evidence of widening, particularly of the proximal and distal radioulnar joints. There should be slight overlapping of the distal radius and ulna at the DRUJ on the anteroposterior projection.

Soft Tissues

Assess all of the soft tissues for any evidence of swelling. On the lateral projection (if an adequate image), occasionally, it might be possible to see a positive sail sign suggesting an elbow joint effusion, which would warrant dedicated projections.

Significant Areas

Assess the radial head and ulna styloid for subtle fractures and the alignment of the proximal and distal radioulnar joint. If you have identified one injury, look for another; remember the ring theory. Consider whether additional projections of the elbow or wrist are needed (either due to the clinical history or because of findings on the forearm radiographs).

Systematic Approach

Radiographic appearances of the forearm (Fig. 4.20)

Anteroposterior and lateral projections

Follow the standard approach to the AABCSS in addition to:

Adequacy	• Are both the elbow and wrist joints included on the image?
	• Do the two projections demonstrate the respective bones and joints at 90° to each other?
	• Is the forearm supinated on AP (radius and ulna not crossed)?
Alignment	• Do the radius and ulna have a slight varus angulation on the AP?
	• Is the radial head articulating with the capitulum (on both projections) – radiocapitellar line (see elbow)?
	• Is there any gross rotation between the elbow and wrist joints?
	• Are the distal radius and ulna superimposed on the lateral?
	• Does the radial angle (see wrist) intersect the head of ulna?
Bones	• Assess the radius and ulna in turn – assess for subtle bumps and steps in cortex, particularly in paediatrics
	• Assess the distal humerus and visible carpal bones at the edge of the images (especially scaphoid)

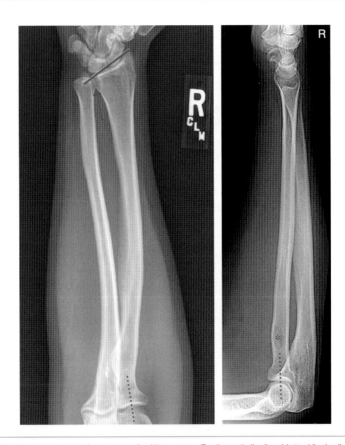

Fig. 4.20 Forearm projections: systematic approach. Alignment – Radiocapitellar line (dotted line), slight varus angulation of radius/ulna, radial angle intersecting head of ulna on AP (solid line), distal radius and ulna superimposed (lateral), wrist and elbow joints grossly aligned. Bones – radius and ulna – assess cortex carefully, particularly in paediatrics; visible carpals and humerus at edge of images. Cartilage – overlap of the distal radius and ulna at the distal radioulnar joint (arrow). Soft tissues – is there any soft tissue swelling? Sail sign in elbow (if true lateral elbow). Significant areas – radial head, neck and styloid; ulna styloid in wrist; alignment of distal and proximal radioulnar joints; do we need dedicated projections of the wrist/elbow? Note the lucency formed by the radial tuberosity (*), which may be mistaken as pathological. (Source: Bontrager's Textbook of Radiographic Positioning and Related Anatomy, Tenth Edition, 2021.)

Cartilage (Joint spaces)	• Is there overlap of distal radius and ulna at distal radioulnar joint (DRUJ) on AP projection? • Not dedicated views, difficult to assess joint spaces • Is there any gross joint space widening of the proximal/distal radioulnar joints?
Soft tissues	• Is there soft tissue swelling? • Are the soft tissue planes displaced? • Is there evidence of an elbow joint effusion (sail sign) on the lateral?
Significant areas	• Look for evidence of radial head, neck, or styloid fracture • Look for evidence of ulna styloid fracture • Assess the alignment of the distal and proximal radioulnar joint • Do we need dedicated elbow/wrist projections?

Fractures/Trauma

 INSIGHT

As a ring structure, a fracture to either the radius or the ulna is usually accompanied by a second, either of the other bone or as a dislocation of either the proximal or distal radioulnar joint.

Forearm Fractures

(Fig. 4.21)

Fractures of both bones in the forearm (without associated joint injury) are relatively common, particularly in paediatrics. Whilst fractures in adults tend to be complete and displaced, in paediatrics, because of the difference in bone composition, fractures may be incomplete or simply bow the bones.

Typical mechanism of injury:
- FOOSH

Clinical presentation:
- May occur in adults and paediatrics
- Localised pain and swelling over forearm

Appearance:
- In adults fractures of both the distal radius and ulna typically occur in the mid/distal forearm and displaced

Fig. 4.21 Forearm fracture. There are displaced fractures of both the mid radius and ulna. It is still important to assess the proximal and distal radioulnar joints for injury. (Source: STATdx © Elsevier.)

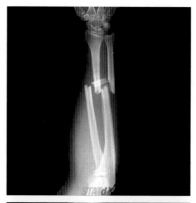

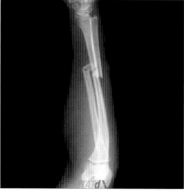

• In paediatrics, dependent on age, fractures may appear bowed, buckled (torus), incomplete (greenstick), or complete

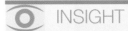

INSIGHT

Because paediatric bones are more elastic than in adults (due to the relative higher proportion of organic to inorganic composition), fractures are often incomplete. The younger the individual, the greater the bone's ability to bow and bend before breaking. As a result, particularly in the forearm and wrist, we see a range of different fracture patterns.

Plastic bowing (Fig. 4.22): Plastic (or elastic) bowing is seen particularly in younger paediatrics. This results in no visible fracture line but smooth and exaggerated bending of the diaphysis of the bones. It is sometimes seen in conjunction with the other types of incomplete fracture below, where the force applied is sufficient to cause an overt fracture as well as the bowing.

Buckle fracture (Fig. 4.23): Sometimes called a *Torus* (ancient Greek for bulge) fracture, as the appearance is of a slight bulging or buckling of the bone cortex on the side of compression, normally dorsal following a FOOSH (think about the force on the wrist). May see two bulges on either side of the bone on the frontal projection.

Often there is no evident fracture line on the opposite (tension) side of the bone, but if there is, then this is usually horizontal and fine and is known as a *lead pipe fracture* (as this is how it breaks if bent!).

Greenstick fracture (Fig. 4.24): Analogy is of bending a young (green) stick. It tends to bend and splinter on one side rather than snap. It is not associated with a bulge on the other cortex (different to a lead pipe fracture).

Fig. 4.22 Plastic bowing. Note the exaggerated curve of the ulna (arrows) without evidence of any fracture line. (Source: STATdx © Elsevier.)

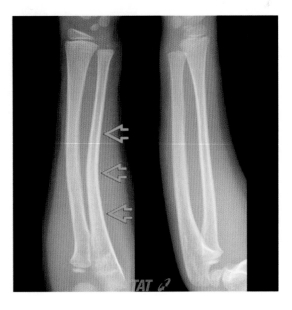

Fig. 4.23 Buckle (torus) fracture. There are very subtle bulges of the medial and lateral cortex of the radius (arrows) and a more obvious buckle on the posterior (compression) aspect (curved arrow) following a FOOSH in this 5-year-old. There is also a very subtle incomplete fracture of the ulna identified by a cortical step (hollow arrow). (Source: STATdx © Elsevier.)

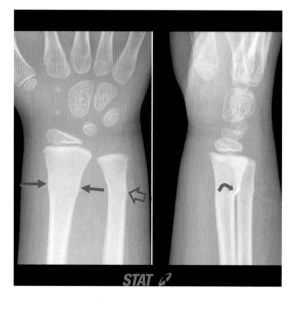

Fig. 4.24 Greenstick fracture. There are incomplete fractures on the anterior (tension) side of both the radius and ulna (hollow arrow) following a FOOSH injury in this 5-year-old. Note that the posterior (compression) side of the cortices (arrows) are intact and not buckled, typical of a greenstick fracture. (Source: STATdx © Elsevier.)

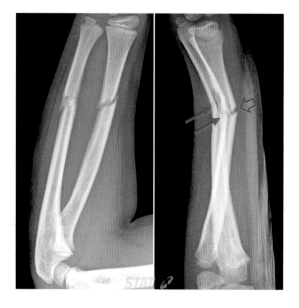

Monteggia Fracture-Dislocation (Fig. 4.25)

First described by Giovanni Monteggia in 1814. Fracture of the proximal shaft (diaphysis) of the ulna with dislocation of the radial head on the capitulum. Relatively rare but often requires surgical intervention. Important to assess radiocapitellar line in any proximal ulna fractures in particular.

Typical mechanism of injury:
- FOOSH with forced pronation (internal rotation of forearm)

Fig. 4.25 Monteggia fracture-dislocation.
There is a displaced fracture of the proximal ulna (arrow) with anterior dislocation of the radial head (hollow arrow). Note the radiocapitellar line (dotted line) does not bisect the capitulum (C). (Source: STATdx © Elsevier.)

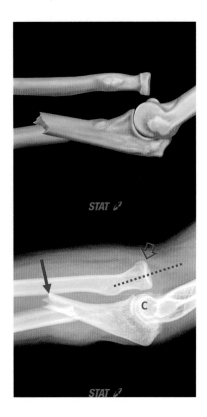

Clinical presentation:
- More common in adults than paediatrics
- Localised pain and swelling over elbow and proximal forearm, restricted movement

Appearance:
- Ulna fracture usually in mid/proximal shaft and obvious due to displacement
- Dislocation of radial head normally anterior and obvious; may be subtle
- Assess radiocapitellar line on elbow/forearm projection; radial head will not articulate with capitulum

Galeazzi Fracture-Dislocation (Figs. 4.26 and 4.40)

First described by Riccardo Galeazzi in 1934. Effectively opposite to Monteggia: fracture of distal shaft of radius with dislocation of head of ulna at DRUJ. High levels of morbidity if dislocation of DRUJ is not managed. Important to assess alignment of DRUJ in any distal radius fractures in particular.

Typical mechanism of injury:
- FOOSH with flexed elbow

Clinical presentation:
- Both paediatrics (typically age 9–12) and adults
- Localised pain and swelling over distal forearm and wrist

Fig. 4.26 Galeazzi fracture-dislocation.
There is a displaced fracture of the distal radius (arrow). There is also dislocation of the DRUJ demonstrated by widening of the joint space (hollow arrow), the radial angle on the AP does not intersect the head of ulna (solid line), and there is lack of superimposition of the head of ulna with the radius on the lateral (dotted line). (Source: STATdx © Elsevier.)

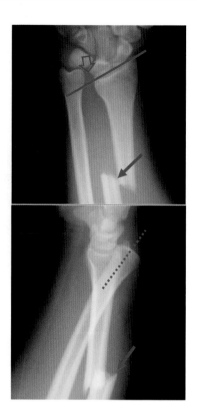

Appearance:
- Ulna fracture usually in mid/distal shaft and obvious due to displacement
- Dislocation of DRUJ often apparent, but look for widening of joint and the radial angle (see page 73) not intersecting the head of ulna on the AP, and lack of superimposition of distal radius and ulna on lateral projection
- In paediatrics, there may be a fracture through the distal ulna physeal plate instead of dislocation of the DRUJ.

Nightstick (or Parry) Fracture

Occasionally an isolated fracture of the ulna can occur without any associated second injury (rules are there to be broken, literally in this case!). This injury is so called for when someone is struck with a 'nightstick' (baton or truncheon) and the arm is raised to protect, or 'parry', the blow. Similar injuries of the radius can occur, though they are less common.

Typical mechanism of injury:
- Direct blow to forearm, such as being struck by a blunt object

Clinical presentation:
- Localised pain over forearm

Appearance:
- Fracture normally of the mid-ulna (rarely radius), may be displaced or undisplaced
- Always check for a second injury

WRIST

Like the elbow, the wrist is a complex structure and can be very challenging to interpret given the number of bones and articulations to consider. Again, a systematic approach for each aspect helps negotiate the complexity, though it can take time to be thorough.

Whilst there are several projections often used to image the wrist (including obliques and scaphoid projections), the main two are the dorsipalmar (DP) and lateral, so we will concentrate on those individually, since there is a lot to consider for each.

As with any radiographic projections, but particularly joints, positioning of the wrist is absolutely essential, and sub-optimal images can considerably affect the relationships and appearances described. The image should also be centred over the wrist joint; a hand/wrist projection is not adequate to evaluate the wrist.

Dorsipalmar Projection

Adequacy

It is important to ensure the wrist is in a neutral position and the hand is not deviated towards either the radial or ulnar side. Changing the position of the hand like this can alter the normal appearances seen, in particular:

- *Scaphoid*; ulna deviation causes elongation of the scaphoid. Whilst this potentially makes scaphoid fractures easier to visualise, it does alter the arrangement of the other carpal bones. Radial deviation causes foreshortening of the scaphoid, which can obscure fractures and also mimic instability and rotation of the scaphoid which can be caused by injury (see Fig. 4.55).
- *Lunate*; when the wrist is in a neutral position, the lunate appears square in shape; radial deviation can cause it to become triangular in appearance, which can mimic injury.

Alignment

There are several lines which can be used to help assess the normal alignment of the wrist joint.

Radial angle (Fig. 4.27): a line drawn from the radial styloid to the medial aspect of its articular surface should normally bisect the head of the ulna. Disruption of the DRUJ due to injury can cause this relationship to be lost, though sometimes normal variants can cause the ulna to be longer or shorter than normal.

Arcs of Gilula (Fig. 4.28): three arcs which relate to the normal alignment of the distal and proximal rows of the carpals. These arcs should be smooth and without steps/interruptions, which might indicate fracture or ligamentous injury. The three arcs are:

First arc: proximal surfaces of the scaphoid, lunate, and triquetrum
Second arc: distal surfaces of scaphoid, lunate, and triquetrum
Third arc: proximal surfaces of capitate and hamate

Fig. 4.27 DP wrist projection: alignment – radial angle. A line drawn through the tip of the radial styloid (R) and medial aspect of the articular surface (arrow) should bisect the head of the ulna (U). (Source: Bontrager's Textbook of Radiographic Positioning and Related Anatomy, Tenth Edition, 2021.)

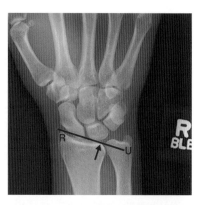

Fig. 4.28 DP wrist projection: alignment – arcs of Gilula. Used to assess carpal alignment and should be smooth. First arc (green) – proximal row of carpals. Second arc (blue) – distal surface of proximal row. Third arc (red) – proximal surface of distal row. (Source: Bontrager's Textbook of Radiographic Positioning and Related Anatomy, Tenth Edition, 2021.)

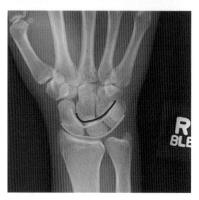

Bones (Fig. 4.29)

It is important to assess each of the visualised bones in turn by looking at their shape, tracing their cortex, and looking at their internal texture, including the distal radius and ulna, all of the carpal bones, and the visualised metacarpals. In particular it is important to consider some specific areas:

- Scaphoid: look very carefully for subtle lucent lines or cortical steps, particularly in the waist and tuberosity.
- Lunate: should appear square in shape (will change if hand not in neutral position or due to injury). The lunate should also normally have more than half of its surface parallel to the distal radius; positioning can also change this alignment.
- Hamate: the hook of hamate is seen as a separate round area within the body. Loss of this circle may indicate a fracture (though rare).
- Base of thumb metacarpal; this is a commonly fractured area and clinically may mimic a scaphoid fracture.

 INSIGHT

A normal variant which is sometimes mistaken for fracture is the remnant of the distal radius physeal plate. When it fuses, it sometimes leaves a fine sclerotic line and a small step (beak) in the lateral cortex (Fig. 4.30).

Fig. 4.29 DP wrist projection: bones. Assess all bones but in particular: scaphoid (red) – look for subtle fractures; lunate (blue) – should be square in shape and more than half should articulate with radius; hamate (green) – look for presence of hook (purple) within body; base of thumb metacarpal (T); radial (R) and ulna (U) styloid processes. (Source: Bontrager's Textbook of Radiographic Positioning and Related Anatomy, Tenth Edition, 2021.)

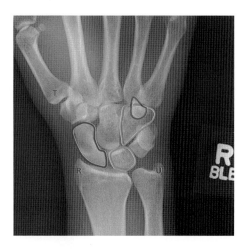

Fig. 4.30 Physeal plate remnant. On the lateral surface of the distal radius (arrow), there is a subtle cortical irregularity, or 'beak,' which should not be mistaken for fracture. (Source: STATdx © Elsevier.)

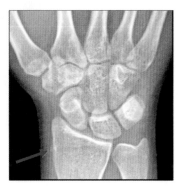

Cartilage (Fig. 4.31)

Intercarpal joint spaces: assess each of the joint spaces between the carpals; these should be uniform in width (1–2 mm) throughout. In particular, assess the *scapholunate distance*, which is relatively commonly widened due to ligamentous injury.

Distal radioulnar joint (DRUJ): there should normally be some minimal overlap (or at least touching) of the distal radius and ulna.

Carpometacarpal (CMC) joints: assess the joint spaces between the bases of the metacarpals and the corresponding carpal(s). There should be uniform joint space for each, though the thumb CMC joint is usually slightly wider.

In paediatrics, also assess the width of the physeal plate of the distal radius and ulna to ensure it is not widened/narrowed.

Look within each joint for the presence of intra-articular bone fragments.

Soft Tissues (Fig. 4.31)

Assess all of the soft tissues for any evidence of swelling.

Scaphoid fat stripe; normally visible lateral to the scaphoid between the trapezium and ulna styloid. Loss of this stripe may indicate fracture (though it is not always reliable).

Fig. 4.31 DP wrist projection: cartilage (joints) and soft tissues.
Cartilage – *CMC joints* (top image; red line): should see a clear joint between each metacarpal and corresponding carpal(s). These joints typically look like a 'zigzag'. *Intercarpal* joints: should be equal and uniform (1–2 mm), in particular scapholunate distance (arrow) between scaphoid (S) and lunate (L). *DRUJ* (hollow arrow): the distal radius and ulna should be slightly overlapping/touching. Soft tissues – soft tissue swelling? Is the scaphoid fat stripe evident (curved arrow)? (Source: STATdx © Elsevier; Bontrager's Textbook of Radiographic Positioning and Related Anatomy, Tenth Edition, 2021.)

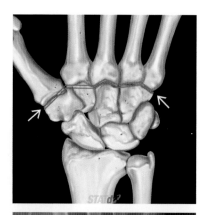

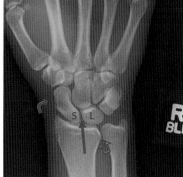

Significant Areas

Assess the scaphoid bone and radial and ulna styloid processes for subtle fractures as well as the integrity of the DRUJ. Make sure you have looked at the radius/ulna and metacarpals right up to the edge of the image.

Systematic Approach

Radiographic appearances of the dorsipalmar wrist (Figs. 4.27–4.29, 4.31)

Dorsipalmar (DP) wrist projection

Follow the standard approach to the AABCSS in addition to:

Adequacy	• Is the wrist in a neutral position and is the hand not deviated to the radial or ulna sides? • Is the image centred over the wrist joint?
Alignment	• Radial angle; does a line drawn along the articular surface intersect the head of ulna? • Are the three lines of Gilula (carpal alignment) smooth?
Bones	• Assess the radius and ulna in turn – assess for subtle bumps and steps in cortex, particularly in paediatrics • Assess each of the carpals in turn • Assess each of the visualised metacarpals

Cartilage (Joint spaces)	• Is there overlap of distal radius and ulna at distal radioulnar joint (DRUJ)?
	• Are the intercarpal joints uniform in width – in particular, assess the scapholunate distance?
	• Assess the CMC joint spaces for uniform width
	• Paediatrics – is the physeal plate of the distal radius/ulna widened/narrowed?
	• Are there any intra-articular bone fragments?
Soft tissues	• Is there soft tissue swelling?
	• Scaphoid fat stripe
Significant areas	• Assess the radial and ulna styloid processes
	• Assess the scaphoid for subtle fractures, particularly the waist
	• Is the lunate square in shape?
	• Is the hook of hamate visible?

Lateral Projection

Adequacy

Ensure the wrist is lateral, with the ulna and radial styloid processes super-imposed. This is important for true assessment of alignment but also for visualising fractures. A rotated lateral (oblique) can demonstrate additional information or help demonstrate further fractures but a true lateral should always be sought.

Fig. 4.32 Lateral wrist projection: alignment – carpals. The normal alignment should be: metacarpals (yellow), sit upon; capitate (blue), sits within; lunate (red), sits upon; distal radius (green). There should be a clear joint space between each.

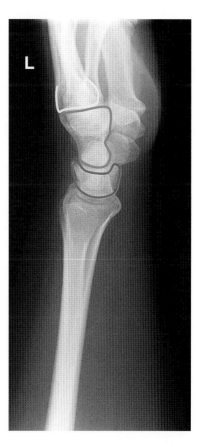

Alignment

Carpal alignment (Fig. 4.32): the visualisation of individual carpal bones on the lateral projection can be quite confusing, and not all bones can be clearly visualised, but the alignment of the wrist is sometimes likened to an apple in a cup on a saucer! The apple (proximal part of capitate) should sit within the cup (lunate), which then sits on the saucer (distal radius). Loss of this normal arrangement indicates injury, usually a dislocation. In addition, the base of the metacarpals should lie on the distal surface of the capitate.

Scaphoid (Fig. 4.33): further to the alignment above, if a line is drawn through the capitate/lunate/radius, then the scaphoid lies at an angle approximately 45° anterior to this line. An increase/decrease in this angle is suggestive of ligamentous injury or instability.

Radial/volar tilt (Fig. 4.34): a line drawn from the posterior (dorsal) to the anterior (volar) parts of the distal radius should normally form an angle of approximately 20° from the horizontal. Reduction in this angle in particular is suggestive of a distal radius fracture, even if a fracture line cannot be visualised.

Fig. 4.33 Lateral wrist projection: alignment – scaphoid. The scaphoid (solid lines) normally lies at an angle of approximately 45° to the line through the lunate/capitate (dotted line).

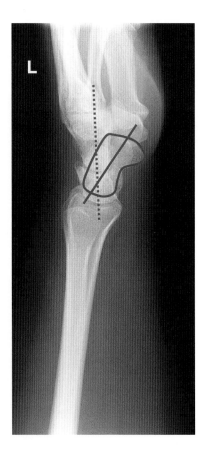

Fig. 4.34 Lateral wrist projection: alignment – radial (volar) tilt. The line between the dorsal and volar aspects of the distal radius (solid line) should be approximately 20° to the horizontal (dotted line).

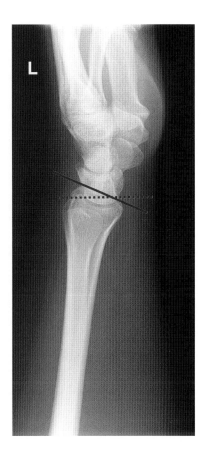

Bones (Fig. 4.35)

As per the DP projection, assess all of the visualised bones (radius/ulna, carpals, and metacarpals). Special attention should be given to the following:

- *Distal radius*: this is a common fracture site. The posterior (dorsal) surface should be smooth and rounded; assess for any step or bulging.
- *Scaphoid*: although most of the scaphoid may be superimposed by other carpals, the distal pole and tuberosity will be visible and should be assessed for subtle fracture.
- *Triquetrum*: assess the posterior surface of the carpal bones for small fragments of bone. Fractures of the triquetrum often demonstrate a small avulsion fracture in this area.
- *Thumb metacarpal*: as on the DP projection, assess the base of thumb metacarpal.

Cartilage (Fig. 4.32)

A clear and uniform joint space should be evident between each of the capitate, lunate, and distal radius.

In paediatrics, assess the width of the physeal plate of the distal radius and ulna to ensure it is not widened/narrowed.

Fig. 4.35 Lateral wrist projection: bones and soft tissues. Bones – assess all bones, but in particular: *distal radius* (R): in particular dorsal surface (arrow); *scaphoid* (S): distal pole; *triquetrum*: assess for bone fragments (hollow arrow); *thumb metacarpal* (T). Soft tissues – pronator fat stripe (dotted line). Should be parallel to volar surface of distal radius.

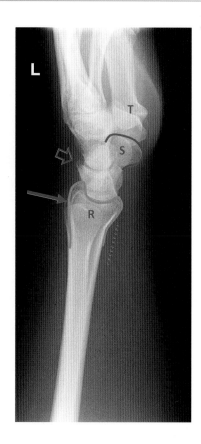

Soft Tissues (Fig. 4.35)   Assess all of the soft tissues for any evidence of swelling. The pronator fat stripe is a plane of fat normally visualised anterior to the distal radius and ulna, between the pronator quadratus and flexor digitorum muscles. Displacement, or loss, of this stripe has been described as being suggestive of injury and, whilst its reliability is questioned, is certainly worthy of a closer inspection of the image.

Significant Areas   Make sure you have looked at the radius/ulna and metacarpals right up to the edge of the image, as well as take another look at the scaphoid and distal radius for very subtle injuries.

Systematic Approach

Radiographic appearances of the lateral wrist (Figs. 4.32–4.35)

Lateral wrist projection

Follow the standard approach to the AABCSS in addition to:

Adequacy	• Are the radial and ulna styloid processes superimposed?
Alignment	• Do the base of metacarpals, capitate, lunate, and distal radius all lie along the same line?
	• Does the scaphoid form a 45° anterior to the line above?
	• Radial tilt; is the line between the posterior and anterior aspect of the distal radius at approximately 20° from the horizontal?

Bones	• Assess the distal radius and ulna in turn – assess for subtle bumps and steps in cortex, particularly in paediatrics
	• Assess each of the visualised carpals in turn, in particular the scaphoid
	• Are there any avulsion fractures posterior (dorsal) to the carpal bones?
	• Assess each of the visualised metacarpals, especially the thumb
Cartilage (Joint spaces)	• Are there uniform joint spaces between the capitate, lunate, and distal radius?
	• Paediatrics – is the physeal plate of the distal radius/ulna widened/narrowed?
Soft tissues	• Is there any soft tissue swelling?
	• Is the pronator fat stipe evident or is it displaced/missing?
Significant areas	• Assess the dorsal cortex of the distal radius for steps/bumps
	• Assess the scaphoid
	• Assess the bones at the edge of the image

Fractures/Trauma

Injuries to the wrist are very common, particularly due to falls. The range of possible injuries (both bone and soft tissue) demonstrated around the wrist too extensive to include in this book, so here we will concentrate on the more commonly encountered.

Some have already been described under the forearm, and others relating to the thumb and CMC joints are covered in the respective parts later in this chapter. The specific wrist injuries covered here can be loosely divided into those that involve the distal radius and ulna and those that involve the carpals.

 INSIGHT

Distal radius fractures are typically referred to by eponyms, though these do offer generalisations of injuries, and often there is variation in the injuries demonstrated compared to the 'classic' description. Many were described before we had X-ray images and so were based upon clinical appearance only! As with all eponyms, they should be used with caution, and a full description of the findings is preferable. One of the key aspects of these injuries is whether the fracture is intra-articular and extends into the radiocarpal joint.

The following injuries will be considered in this chapter:

Distal radius/ulna fractures:
- Colles
- Smith (reverse Colles)
- Radial styloid (Hutchinson/chauffeurs)
- Barton (and reverse Barton) fracture
- Diepunch fracture
- Salter-Harris II
- Ulna styloid fractures (can occur alone but commonly with distal radius fractures)

Carpal fractures:
- Scaphoid
- Triquetrum

Carpal dislocations/soft tissue injuries:
- Perilunate dislocation
- Mid-carpal dislocation
- Lunate dislocation
- Scapholunate dissociation

Distal Radius Fractures

Colles Fracture
(Figs. 4.36 and 4.37)

First described by Abraham Colles in 1814 (90 years before X-rays were discovered!). Described as a transverse fracture of the distal radial metaphysis with posterior/dorsal angulation and/or displacement. They are often associated with an avulsion fracture of the ulna styloid. Very common injury.

Typical mechanism of injury:
- FOOSH; compression on dorsal aspect, tension on volar aspect.

Clinical presentation:
- Adults over the age of 40; females more commonly than men
- More common in patients with osteoporosis
- Pain and swelling of distal radius
- 'Dinner fork' deformity due to angulation of fracture

Appearance:
- Transverse fracture of distal radius within the metaphysis (proximal to joint), often involves some impaction of fracture
- May be subtle if minimally displaced; assess volar tilt (which will be reduced/reversed) and posterior cortex of distal radius
- Assess for dorsal/posterior displacement and angulation
- Avulsion fracture of ulna styloid common
- Normally no extension of fracture into wrist joint (extra-articular)

Fig. 4.36 Colles fracture; left wrist. The transverse fracture of the metaphysis is seen anteriorly (arrow), and there is impaction dorsally (hollow arrow). Dorsal (posterior) angulation is demonstrated, and there is reversal of the normal volar tilt (dotted line) compared to Fig. 4.34. Note how the appearance of the shape of the wrist resembles a fork and the fracture does not extend into the wrist joint. (Source: STATdx © Elsevier.)

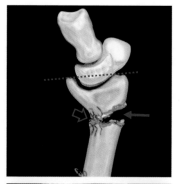

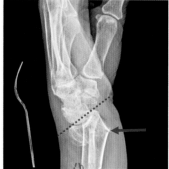

Fig. 4.37 Colles fracture; right wrist. There is a sclerotic appearance of the distal radial metaphysis on the DP projection due to impaction of the fracture (*). There is loss of the normal volar tilt of the radius (dotted line) and convexity of the dorsal surface (hollow arrow) on the lateral projection. Note the commonly associated ulna styloid fracture (curved arrow), and there is displacement of the pronator fat stripe (straight arrow). (Source: STATdx © Elsevier.)

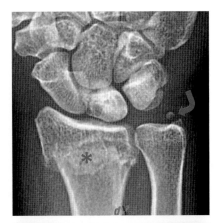

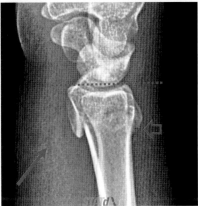

Smith's (Reverse Colles) Fracture

(Fig. 4.38)

Described by Robert Smith in 1847. Transverse fracture of the distal radial metaphysis with anterior/volar displacement and/or angulation; effectively the opposite appearance of a Colles fracture.

Typical mechanism of injury:

- Fall onto dorsal aspect of hand/forced flexion of wrist, such as a fall when carrying a shopping bag
- Less common due to mechanism of injury

Clinical presentation:

- Pain, swelling, and deformity of wrist
- Less association with a particular age

Appearance:

- Transverse fracture of distal radius within the metaphysis (proximal to joint), often involves some impaction of fracture
- May be subtle if minimally displaced; assess volar tilt, which may be increased
- Assess for volar/anterior displacement and angulation
- Normally no extension of fracture into wrist joint (extra-articular)

Fig. 4.38 Smith (reverse Colles) fracture. There is a fracture through the distal radial metaphysis (hollow arrows) with volar/anterior displacement (arrow) – the reverse of what is seen in a Colles fracture. Note the soft tissue swelling. (Source: STATdx © Elsevier.)

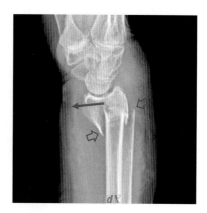

Radial Styloid Fracture (Figs. 4.39 and 4.40)

Also known as *Hutchinson* (described by Jonathan Hutchinson in 1866) or *chauffeur* fracture; so called as it was seen following injury where a car back-fired when being hand-started and the crank compressed the wrist. Described as oblique fractures of the radial styloid which extend into the wrist joint. Often associated with carpal ligament injury and displacement.

Typical mechanism of injury:
- FOOSH; compression causes scaphoid to transmit force through radial styloid
- Direct blow on radial styloid
- Rarely seen in chauffeurs today!

Clinical presentation:
- Pain and swelling of wrist

Appearance:
- Oblique fracture of radial styloid
- Intra-articular; extension into radiocarpal joint
- Assess carpal arcs and scapholunate distance (in particular) for associated injury

Fig. 4.39 Radial styloid fracture. There is an oblique fracture of the radial styloid, extending into the radiocarpal joint (arrow). The carpal arcs and intercarpal distances are normal. Associated soft tissue injury to the wrist is fairly common. Continued in Fig. 4.40. (Source: STATdx © Elsevier.)

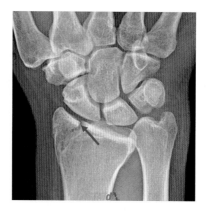

Fig. 4.40 Radial styloid fracture and Galeazzi injury. Same case as Fig. 4.39. Note on the DP that the radial angle (dotted line) does not intersect the head of ulna (U). The lateral demonstrates clear disruption of the DRUJ and warranted projections of the forearm (not included), which demonstrated a fracture of the shaft of radius; consistent with a Galeazzi injury. (Source: STATdx © Elsevier.)

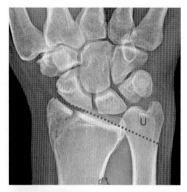
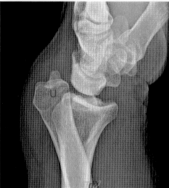

Barton (Fig. 4.41) and Reverse Barton
(Figs. 4.42 and 4.43)
Fracture

First described by John Barton in 1838. Both are intra-articular fractures of the distal radius which extend into the radial carpal joint. The fracture fragment and carpals displace together, causing a dislocation of the wrist too. Barton fracture involves a fracture of the dorsal surface of the distal radius with dorsal displacement. The reverse Barton is a fracture of the volar surface with volar displacement.

The intra-articular component of these fractures helps distinguish them from Colles and Smith fractures.

Typical mechanism of injury:
- Barton: similar to Colles – FOOSH but particularly if wrist is pronated (such as falling backwards onto an eternally rotated arm, e.g. when snowboarding)
- Reverse Barton: similar to Smith – fall onto dorsal aspect of hand

Clinical presentation:
- Either in paediatrics (typically around puberty) or in older adults
- Wrist pain, swelling, and deformity

Appearance:
- Fracture of dorsal surface of distal radius (Barton) with dorsal displacement of carpals at radiocarpal joint. Loss of volar tilt of the radius
- Fracture of volar surface of distal radius (reverse Barton) with volar displacement of carpals at radiocarpal joint
- Assess for intra-articular extension of fracture into wrist joint (helps differentiate from Colles/Smith fractures)

Fig. 4.41 Barton fracture; right wrist.
There is an intra-articular fracture through the dorsal surface of the distal radius (hollow arrow) with dorsal dislocation (arrows) of the carpal bones which are still articulating with the fracture fragment. The involvement of the radiocarpal joint, and that it is more distal, distinguishes this injury from a Colles fracture. Note the air in the soft tissues (curved arrows) indicating this in an open fracture. (Source: STATdx © Elsevier.)

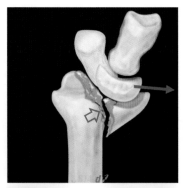

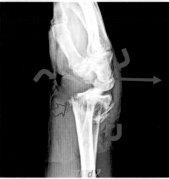

Fig. 4.42 Reverse Barton fracture; right wrist.
In contrast to Fig 4.41, there is an intra-articular fracture through the volar surface of the distal radius (hollow arrows) with volar dislocation (arrows) of the carpal bones which are still articulating with the fracture fragment. The involvement of the radiocarpal joint, and that it is more distal, distinguishes this injury from a Smith fracture. (Source: STATdx © Elsevier.)

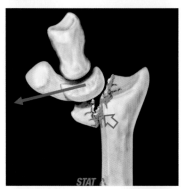

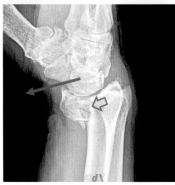

Fig. 4.43 Reverse Barton fracture. Same case as Fig. 4.42, this sagittal CT image clearly demonstrates the intra-articular fracture (arrow) of the volar surface of the distal radius. (Source: STATdx © Elsevier.)

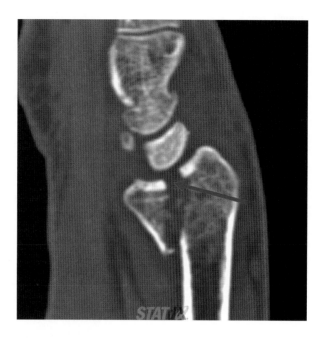

Diepunch Fractures

(Figs. 4.44 and 4.45)

Axial compression of the carpals (scaphoid and lunate) into the distal radius articular surface effectively 'punches out' a fracture, hence the name. Classically causes comminuted fracture in both the sagittal and coronal planes of the distal radius with a depressed fragment where the scaphoid and lunate articulate. May be associated with fractures of scaphoid/lunate, carpal and DRUJ disruption, and fractures of the ulna styloid. Often require CT for full evaluation due to complexity of injury.

Typical mechanism of injury:
- FOOSH; axial compression of carpals into articular surface of radius

Clinical presentation:
- Wrist pain, swelling, and deformity
- Low-energy trauma in older adults with osteoporosis, higher energy in young adults

Appearance:
- Range from very subtle to very obvious on radiographs
- Comminuted intra-articular fracture involving the articular surface of the distal radius
- Depressed fragment of distal radius
- Loss of volar tilt of radius
- Assess articular surface of radius for any cortical steps/interruptions
- Assess DRUJ for disruption; widening of DRUJ, radial angle does not bisect head of ulna
- Look for associated fractures of ulna styloid, scaphoid, and lunate
- Assessment of carpal arcs and intercarpal spaces for possible disruption

Fig. 4.44 Diepunch fracture. This fracture on the DP radiograph demonstrates a very subtle depression/irregularity (arrow) in the cortex of the articular surface of the radius. The coronal CT shows more clearly the fracture (hollow arrow) caused by the scaphoid 'punching out' the articular surface of the radius. Note also the apparent widening of the scapholunate distance (curved arrows) compared to the other intercarpal joints, suggestive of injury to the scapholunate ligament. (Source: STATdx © Elsevier.)

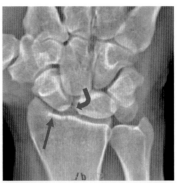

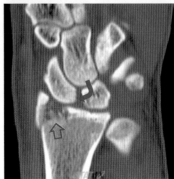

Fig. 4.45 Diepunch fracture. This not so subtle injury has caused intra-articular fractures of the distal radius in the sagittal plane (arrow) splitting the radius into medial and lateral fragments, and in the coronal plane (hollow arrow) splitting the radius into volar and dorsal components. The force of the carpals compressing the articular surface of the radius has caused it to split into four main parts (and some other smaller fragments besides). Note the ulna styloid fracture but there is no disruption of the carpal arcs. (Source: STATdx © Elsevier.)

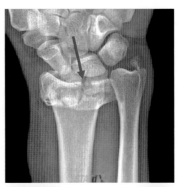

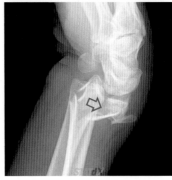

Salter-Harris II Fractures (Fig. 4.46)

Only occurring in paediatrics (prior to closure of the distal radius physeal plate); whilst other Salter-Harris fractures are possible, the type II injury is most common. This type of fracture causes a cartilage fracture through the physeal plate as well as a bone fracture more proximally though the metaphysis.

Typical mechanism of injury:
- FOOSH

Clinical presentation:
- Typically paediatrics aged 8–16 prior to closure of physeal plate
- Pain, swelling, and deformity of wrist

Appearance:
- Lateral projection; widening of the physeal plate, posterior displacement of the epiphysis, loss of volar tilt of radius
- Fracture fragment from the dorsal metaphysis of the distal radius, still attached to epiphysis; size may vary
- Subtle injuries may be difficult to identify on the DP projection. In significant injuries it is also often not possible to identify the involvement of the fracture fragment and involvement of the physeal plate
- Associated ulna styloid fractures common

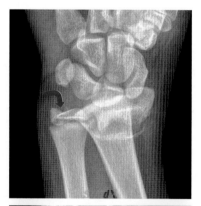
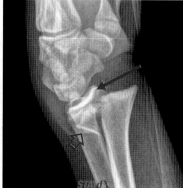

Fig. 4.46 Salter-Harris II fracture; left wrist. The DP projection shows an abnormality of the distal radius but not how the physeal plate is involved. The lateral demonstrates there is posterior displacement of the radial epiphysis (arrow) indicating a fracture of the physeal plate. There is also a large triangular fracture fragment (hollow arrow) from the dorsal aspect of the radius. The combination of these two indicates a Salter-Harris II fracture. Note there is an associated fracture of the ulna styloid (curved arrow). (Source: STATdx © Elsevier.)

Carpal Fractures

Scaphoid fractures make up approximately 70% of all carpal injuries, followed by the triquetrum (~15%). Other fractures are rare and often associated with other fractures or dislocations, and so thorough systematic approach is required.

Scaphoid Fracture

(Figs. 4.47 and 4.48)

We could write a whole chapter about scaphoid fractures, but we won't! The scaphoid is the most commonly fractured carpal and one of the most commonly fractured bones in the body. Whilst the majority are minimally displaced and heal without complication, approximately 10% lead to non-union and/or osteonecrosis. Because the scaphoid is considered a bridge between the proximal and distal carpal rows, fracture can also lead to instability. As a consequence, early and accurate diagnosis and treatment are essential to reduce the chance of complications, loss of function, and morbidity.

 INSIGHT

The majority (over 80%) of the blood supply to the scaphoid enters through the waist. The mid and proximal parts are almost entirely supplied by this branch, though the distal pole has supplementary and separate supply which enters distally (so less affected). Fractures through the waist and proximal poles can interrupt this main supply, which either delays or prevents healing (*delayed or non-union*), or causes the proximal part of the bone to die – *osteonecrosis* (Fig. 4.47).

Fig. 4.47 Scaphoid; blood supply and fracture location. The blood supply of the scaphoid enters distally and then perfuses each of the regions of the scaphoid. For this reason, fractures through the waist (B) or proximal pole (C) potentially cuts off the blood supply to the proximal parts (in blue) and lead to osteonecrosis. Fractures though the distal pole (A) do not normally suffer this complication, as the blood supply is normally not interrupted, since it also has a small separate supply. (Source: STATdx © Elsevier.)

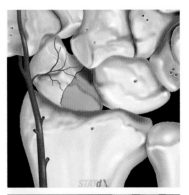

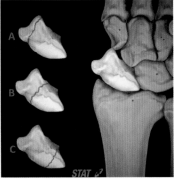

Fig. 4.48 Scaphoid fractures. (A) Some scaphoid fractures (arrow) are displaced and do not cause a diagnostic dilemma, though displaced waist fractures like this may lead to delayed/non-union and osteonecrosis. **(B)** is an initial DP radiograph which demonstrates a subtle cortical step (arrow) though no clear fracture line. **(C)** is the same case but taken 10 days later after immobilisation. The cortical step (arrow) is more apparent, and there is subtle increased lucency within the waist of the scaphoid (hollow arrow) compared to the distal and proximal parts. Early healing leads to bone resorption around the fracture site, which makes the fracture more visible. (Source: STATdx © Elsevier.)

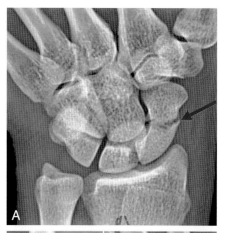
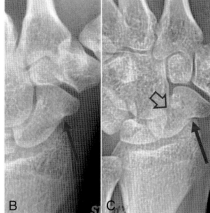

Imaging plays a significant role in the diagnosis of scaphoid fractures. Whilst radiographs remain the initial modality of choice, some scaphoid fractures may be very subtle, visible on only one projection, or even occult.

If initial radiographs are normal, and fracture is still suspected, then wrist immobilisation and follow-up imaging are normally required. MRI is considered the modality of choice, though CT is also widely utilised.

Delayed radiographs of the scaphoid (after 10–14 days) may show evidence of early healing and increased fracture detection and, as well as nuclear medicine bone scans, are also potential alternative imaging methods; however, their use is less common than previously.

Typical mechanism of injury:
- FOOSH; dorsiflexion and radial deviation
- Compression along scaphoid, proximal pole trapped between capitate and radius

Clinical presentation:
- Young adults (16–40 years) after closure of radial physeal plate
- Tenderness over anatomical snuff box; natural hollow at base of thumb

Appearance:
- Best visualised on DP, pronated (AP) oblique, and DP with ulna deviation (scaphoid projections)
- Poor positioning, such as DP in radial deviation, can obscure fractures
- Displaced fractures usually clearly evident
- Subtle fractures; cortical and trabecular disruption, fine lucent lines transverse/oblique to long axis of scaphoid
- Approximate distribution of fracture location:
  - Tubercle – 5%
  - Distal pole – 15%
  - Middle 1/3 (waist) – 70%
  - Proximal pole – 10%
- Assessment of other review areas essential as commonly associated with other wrist injuries

Triquetral Fracture
(Fig. 4.49)

Second most commonly fractured carpal bone.
Typical mechanism of injury:
- FOOSH; axial force on dorsiflexed wrist causing triquetrum to become compressed between hamate and ulna
- Often associated with perilunate dislocations

Clinical presentation:
- Focal tenderness over dorsum of wrist, swelling, and weakness when gripping

Appearance:
- Best seen on lateral projection as fracture fragment over dorsal aspect of carpals
- Overlying soft tissue swelling
- Only larger fractures of the body likely to be demonstrated on DP projection
- Assess carpal alignment due to association with perilunate dislocation

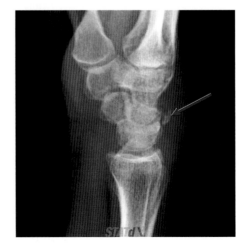

Fig. 4.49 Triquetral fracture. The small bony fragment (arrow) overlying the dorsal aspect of the carpals is the classic appearance of the triquetral fracture. Note the soft tissue swelling. Normal carpal alignment should be assessed, as there is an association between triquetral fractures and perilunate dislocation. (Source: STATdx © Elsevier.)

Carpal Dislocations/Soft Tissue Injuries

As well as fractures, the wrist is prone to dislocations and soft tissue injuries, such as ligamentous tears. Commonly fractures are associated with such injuries, so it is important we use our satisfaction of search to assess for their presence, and whilst on radiographs soft tissue injuries are not necessarily visible, we can use the alignment, joint spaces, and soft tissue planes to help identify them.

Previously in this chapter we discussed the alignment of the carpals by assessing the carpal arcs and shape of the lunate on the DP projection (Figs. 4.28 and 4.29), and the co-axial arrangement on the lateral projection between the capitate, lunate, and distal radius (Fig. 4.32); remember the apple in the cup in the saucer.

There is a progressive 'spectrum' of injuries (Fig. 4.50) that will be considered here but all have similar mechanisms of injury and clinical presentation.

Fig. 4.50 Carpal dislocations. 1 – perilunate dislocation. The capitate (C) is dislocated dorsally, but the lunate (L) remains in articulation with the radius (R). **2** – midcarpal dislocation. The capitate (C) is dislocated dorsally and the lunate (L) rotates and subluxes volarly (anteriorly) but remains in partial articulation with the radius (R). **3** – lunate dislocation. Dislocation of the capitate (C) causes the lunate (L) to dislocate volarly so that it is no longer in articulation with the radius (R). The capitate then migrates proximally to fill the space vacated by the lunate. (Source: STATdx © Elsevier.)

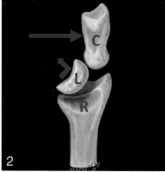

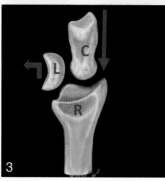

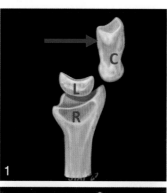

Typical mechanism of injury:
- Axial loading causes hyperextension, supination (internal rotation), and ulna deviation
- Usually high energy, for example, road traffic collisions, falls from height, sports injury

Clinical presentation:
- Focal tenderness, swelling, and deformity
- May present with neuropathy and loss of function due to associated nerve and soft tissue injury
- Perilunate and midcarpal dislocations are more common (but less significant in terms of severity) than lunate dislocations, which are less common (but more significant)

Perilunate Dislocation (Figs. 4.50 and 4.51)

The first stage of the carpal dislocation spectrum is where the capitate (and remaining distal carpals) dislocates dorsally (posteriorly) from its normal position in the lunate: 'the apple falls out of the teacup'. The lunate remains in articulation with the distal radius.

Fig. 4.51 Perilunate dislocation. On the lateral projection the capitate (C) and the remaining carpals are dislocated dorsally, but the lunate (L) remains in articulation with the radius (R). On the DP, the abnormality is more subtle, but the lunate (L, solid line) is less square in shape, and the 2nd carpal arc (dotted line) in particular is disrupted due to the dislocation of the capitate (C) and other carpals on the lunate. (Source: STATdx © Elsevier.)

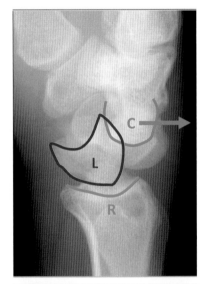

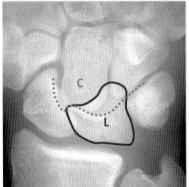

Appearance:

- *DP projection:* disruption of the carpal arcs. Lunate may appear slightly less square in shape than normal due to slight volar rotation (though still articulates with radius)
- *Lateral projection:* capitate (and other carpals) dislocated posteriorly from within the lunate. Lunate may rotate slightly anteriorly though still remain in articulation with distal radius

Midcarpal Dislocation (Figs. 4.50 and 4.52)

Similar to perilunate dislocation, but there is further volar rotation of the lunate, which causes some subluxation (partial dislocation) from the distal radius.

Appearance:

- *DP projection:* disruption of the carpal arcs. Lunate appears more triangular in shape due to volar rotation (though still articulates with radius).
- *Lateral projection:* capitate (and other carpals) dislocated posteriorly from within the lunate. Lunate rotates slightly volarly, and there is some loss of apposition and widening between the articular surfaces of the lunate and distal radius.

Fig. 4.52 Midcarpal dislocation. On the lateral projection the capitate (C) and the remaining carpals are dislocated dorsally. Now the lunate (L) is rotated and subluxed volarly, though it is still partly articulating with the radius (R). On the DP, the abnormality is more subtle, but the lunate (L, solid line) is now triangular in shape. The first and second carpal arcs (dotted lines) are now disrupted due to the dislocation of the capitate (C) and rotation of the lunate. (Source: STATdx © Elsevier.)

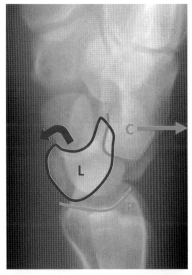

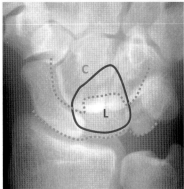

Lunate Dislocation
(Figs. 4.50 and 4.53)

Continuous from the midcarpal dislocation, the lunate continues to rotate anteriorly and then dislocates completely from the distal radius. This leaves a 'void' in the proximal row of carpals between the scaphoid and triquetrum; the capitate displaces proximally to fill this.

> *Appearance:*
> - *DP projection:* disruption of the carpal arcs. Lunate and capitate superimposed and difficult to differentiate. Void between scaphoid and triquetrum may be partially filled by capitate, which displaces proximally.
> - *Lateral projection:* lunate rotated 90° volarly and dislocated to lie anterior to other carpals and radius/ulna. Capitate (and other distal carpals) displaced proximally to lie in closer apposition to distal radius than normal.

Carpal Fracture-Dislocations (Fig. 4.54)

In addition to pure carpal dislocations, additional bony fractures are also seen and are often more common than pure dislocations. When named, the type of dislocation is preceded by the fractured bone with the prefix 'trans-'.

For example, a midcarpal dislocation which also demonstrates a fracture of the radius and scaphoid is named a *transradial transscaphoid midcarpal fracture-dislocation.*

Fig. 4.53 Lunate dislocation. On the lateral projection the lunate (L) is now rotated and dislocated volarly with no articulation with the radius (R). This is called the 'spilled teacup' sign. The capitate (C) now displaces proximally with the remaining carpals to fill the void left by the lunate. On the DP, there is now a void (*) where the lunate (L; solid line) has dislocated from the radius and superimposes with the capitate (C), so they are hard to distinguish. (Source: STATdx © Elsevier.)

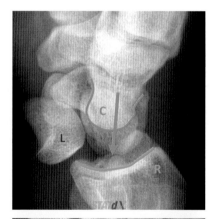

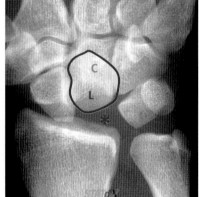

Fig. 4.54 Complex carpal fracture dislocation. The DP projection demonstrates a comminuted scaphoid fracture (arrow) and small fracture fragments adjacent to the capitate (C) and lunate (L). The lunate has more of a triangular appearance, and the carpal arcs, if followed, are disrupted. On the lateral projection the capitate is dislocated dorsally on the lunate, which is rotated and subluxed volarly on the radius (R). The fracture fragments (hollow arrow) are also visible again, apparently from the capitate. This injury combined is known as a trans-scaphoid trans-capitate midcarpal fracture-dislocation. Quite a mouthful! (Source: STATdx © Elsevier.)

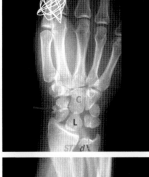
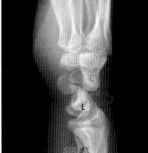

Scapholunate Dissociation (Fig. 4.55)

As well as carpal dislocations, ligamentous rupture of the intercarpal ligaments (and others around the wrist) also occurs following injury. The most common is of the scapholunate ligament, which traverses the joint in between the scaphoid and lunate. Rupture of this ligament causes widening of the joint between these bones, which is visible on radiographs. The gap caused was previously known as the 'Terry Thomas' sign, named after Terry Thomas, who was a 20th-century comedian with a prominent gap between his front teeth.

It may also cause volar rotation of the scaphoid, which appears foreshortened and demonstrates the '*signet ring*' sign due to the distal pole becoming superimposed over the remainder of the bone.

This injury is known as scapholunate dissociation, or diastasis (widening). As with other wrist injuries, this may also occur in conjunction with other concomitant injuries, so, as always, a systematic approach is required.

Typical mechanism of injury:
- FOOSH; hyperextension of wrist with ulna deviation
- May also be chronic rather than post-acute injury and a cause of wrist pain and instability

Clinical presentation:
- Wrist pain and click, especially on radial deviation

Appearance:
- Widening of the scapholunate distance (typically over 3 mm) compared to other intercarpal joints on DP projection – 'Terry Thomas' sign
- Assess for shortening of scaphoid and 'signet ring' sign within scaphoid on DP projection
- Assess both DP and lateral projections for signs of other bone or soft tissue abnormality

Fig. 4.55 Scapholunate dissociation/diastasis.
Compared to the other intercarpal joints, there is marked widening of the scapholunate distance (arrow), in keeping with rupture of the scapholunate ligament which spans the space between the scaphoid (S) and lunate (L). Note also the extra ring structure within the scaphoid compared to Fig. 4.29. Known as the 'signet ring' sign, this indicates volar rotation of the scaphoid which can be due to carpal instability, or by radial deviation of the wrist due to sub-optimal positioning. (Source: STATdx © Elsevier.)

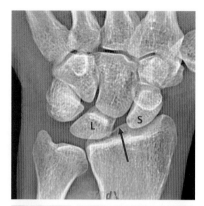

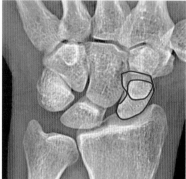

HAND

The hand appears complex because there is a lot to look at, but it can be broken down into predominantly a lot of long bones and joints, and we just need to take time to assess each one – systematically (you may have noticed a theme by now)!

Adequacy

Hand radiographs provide an adequate overview of the skeletal structures in this area but should not replace dedicated projections of the wrist/thumb/finger where clinical indications require them. As part of the systematic approach, you will assess these structures but should interpret them with caution, and dedicated projections may be required if there is suspicion of injury.

It is important to ensure the full area of interest is included, from the distal soft tissues of the fingers and thumb down to the distal radius and ulna.

Alignment

Ensure each of the metacarpophalangeal (MCP) and interphalangeal (IP) joints are aligned on all projections.

On the DP projection the carpal arcs of the wrist, the radial angle intersecting the ulna head, and the integrity of the DRUJ (Figs. 4.27 and 4.28) should be assessed for gross continuity, though remember: these are not dedicated projections and so should be interpreted with caution.

On the oblique and lateral projections, the dorsal surface of the index to little (2nd to 4th) metacarpals should align with the dorsal aspect of the carpals. The thumb metacarpal should articulate with the trapezium. On the lateral projection, the base of metacarpals, capitate, lunate, and distal radius should be in alignment (Fig. 4.32).

Bones

Assess each bone in turn: phalanges, metacarpals, carpals, and distal radius and ulna. Get into a habit of looking at each in turn; for example:

- Start at the tip of the thumb and then assess proximally along each phalanx and metacarpal
- Progress through the index to little fingers in the same way
- Assess the carpals in the same order you would the wrist, for example, along the distal and the proximal rows
- Look at the distal radius and then ulna

For each bone, follow the cortex looking for steps/interruptions and then the internal trabecular pattern for disruption and lucent/sclerotic lines. Look at the overall shape for any angulations (particularly the metacarpals).

Assess the length of the index to little (2nd to 4th) metacarpals; normally the middle finger (3rd) metacarpal should be the longest, followed by the index (2nd), ring (4th), and little (5th). Sometimes the relative lengths of the index and middle metacarpal are interchangeable. You are looking to see gross change in length compared to normal.

Cartilage

As with the bones, take time to look at each joint in a similar way: distal/proximal IP and MCP joints of each digit in turn looking for widening or narrowing of each joint (may indicate subluxation/dislocation) and the presence of small intra-articular bone fragments, particularly in the fingers.

On the DP projection the spaces between the bases of the metacarpals should be assessed for widening/loss. Between the thumb to ring metacarpals (1st to 4th) it is normal to see a slight joint space between the metacarpal bases, but there is normally a slight overlap between the ring and little (4th and 5th) metacarpals.

Also on the DP projection in particular, assess the CMC joint spaces in a similar way to that described in the wrist. The divergence of the X-ray beam in this instance will mean they may not be as clear; assess on the other projections if there is concern.

Soft Tissues

Check for general soft tissue swelling on each projection. If there is soft tissue swelling (sign of injury), assess the adjacent area of bone/joint.

Foreign bodies are also fairly common in the hand, especially with soft tissue lacerations which may be caused by crush and other types of injuries. Look for the presence of air within the soft tissues, especially where fractures are present (in particular the end of the digits), which might indicate they are open.

Significant Areas

There are many common fracture areas in the hand, and whilst the previously systematic approach should have identified them, reviewing them again at the end is useful. These include the head of the index (2nd) and neck of little finger (5th) metacarpals, the base of the proximal phalanges (especially in paediatrics), and the base of the ring and little (4th and 5th) metacarpals/CMC joints.

There may also be overlap in clinical presentation between hand, wrist, and thumb, so it is worth assessing the base of thumb metacarpal, scaphoid, and radial/ulna styloids.

Systematic Approach

Radiographic appearances of the hand (Figs. 4.56 and 4.57)

Hand projections; DP/oblique/lateral

Follow the standard approach to the AABCSS in addition to:

Adequacy	• Are we imaging the correct area? Do we need dedicated finger/thumb/wrist projections? • Are the soft tissues of the digits and distal radius and ulna included? • DP: are the digits extended and joints clear? • Oblique: is it sufficiently different to the DP? • Lateral: are the digits and metacarpals superimposed?
Alignment	• Is each of the IP and MCP joints aligned? • Does the thumb align with the trapezium? • DP: assess the carpal arcs; does the radial angle intersect the head of ulna? Is the DRUJ aligned? • Lateral/oblique: do the dorsal surfaces of the 2nd to 4th CMC joints and the carpals align? • Lateral: do the base of the metacarpals, capitate, lunate, and distal radius align?

Bones	• Assess each bone in turn looking for cortical steps/bumps, internal lucent/sclerotic lines, and assess the shape. Follow:
	  • Tip of thumb phalanx, proximal phalanx, metacarpal
	  • Repeat for index to little fingers
	  • Assess each carpal in turn; distal then proximal row
	  • Assess distal radius and ulna
	 • Assess 2nd to 5th metacarpal length; middle (3rd) should be longest
	 • Are there any sesamoid bones present? Do they look round, smooth, and adjacent to a joint?

Cartilage (Joint spaces)	• Assess each joint space for narrowing/widening and presence of intra-articular bone fragments
	  • Distal and proximal IP and MCP joints; thumb to little finger
	  • Spaces between bases of metacarpals; expect overlap between ring and little (4th and 5th).
	  • Assess CMC joint spaces; are they visible?

Soft tissues	• Is there any soft tissue swelling? • Are there any foreign bodies? • Are there any soft tissue lacerations/air?
Significant areas	• Head of index (2nd) and neck of little finger (5th) metacarpal • Base of proximal phalanges • Base of ring/little (4th/5th) metacarpals • Scaphoid • Radial/ulna styloid processes

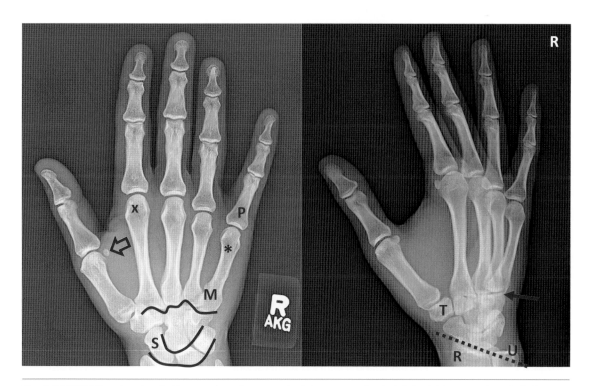

Fig. 4.56 DP/oblique hand projections: systematic approach. Adequacy – extended digits, joint spaces clear; inclusion of distal soft tissues and radius/ulna. Alignment – IP and MCP joints, base of thumb with trapezium (T); DP only, carpal arcs (solid lines); oblique, alignment of base of metacarpals with carpals at CMC joints (arrow); radial angle intersects head of ulna (dotted line). Bones – each digit in turn, phalanges and metacarpals; carpals, distal radius/ulna; any sesamoids? (hollow arrow). Cartilage – joint spaces, IP and MCP joints; DP only, intermetacarpal spaces and CMC joint spaces (zigzag); any intra-articular bone fragments? Soft tissues – is there any soft tissue swelling? Assess bone adjacent to it if present. Any foreign bodies or soft tissue lacerations? Significant areas – head of index (2nd) (x) and neck of little finger (5th) (*) metacarpals; base of proximal phalanges (P) and metacarpals (M); scaphoid (S); radial (R) and ulna (U) styloid processes. (Source: Bontrager's Textbook of Radiographic Positioning and Related Anatomy, Tenth Edition, 2021)

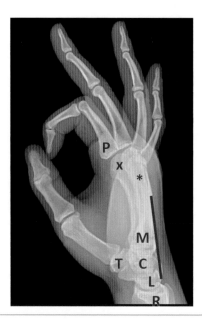

Fig. 4.57 Lateral hand projection: systematic approach. Alignment – IP and MCP joints, base of thumb with trapezium (T); dorsal aspect of metacarpals with dorsal aspect of carpals (solid line); base of metacarpal (M) with capitate (C), lunate (L), and distal radius (R). Bones – each digit in turn, phalanges and metacarpals; carpals, distal radius/ulna; cartilage – joint spaces – IP and MCP joints, thumb CMC joint; any intra-articular bone fragments? Soft tissues – is there any soft tissue swelling? Assess bone adjacent to it if present; any foreign bodies or soft tissue lacerations? Significant areas – head of index (x) and neck of little finger (*) metacarpals; base of proximal phalanges (P) and metacarpals (M); radial and ulna styloid processes. (Source: STATdx © Elsevier.)

Fractures

Hand injuries occur due to a wide range of mechanisms and are considered extremely important to diagnose early, since delayed management can lead to significant functional morbidity and loss of function. Joint involvement and degree of displacement/rotation have important roles to play in the outcome.

Oblique and spiral fractures of the shafts of the metacarpals are fairly easy to identify due to displacement (Fig. 4.58). Rotation at the fracture site, particularly in spiral fractures, is important to identify but is normally better assessed clinically than radiologically.

Boxer's Fracture
(Fig. 4.59)

The name of the injury is perhaps something of a misnomer, since it is rare to see it in professional/trained boxers or fighters. It is more commonly seen as the result of a punch injury in untrained fighters, so perhaps it might be better named the 'scrapper' or 'brawler' fracture.

The injury is described as an oblique fracture through the neck of the little finger (5th) metacarpal with volar angulation of the fracture. The degree of angulation is important in deciding whether management is surgical or conservative. The ring finger (4th) metacarpal is slightly less commonly affected; however, sometimes both are affected simultaneously.

Fig. 4.58 Metacarpal shaft fracture. This is a spiral fracture of the shaft of the ring (4th) metacarpal with slight medial and proximal displacement of the fracture (arrow). (Source: STATdx © Elsevier.)

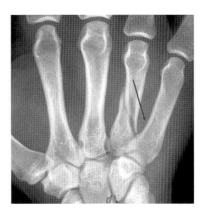

Fig. 4.59 Boxer's fracture. (A) demonstrates the classic appearance of this type of injury, an oblique fracture of the neck of the little finger (5th) metacarpal with volar angulation of the head (arrow). There is adjacent soft tissue swelling. Healed fractures result in a persistent angulation unless manipulated and reduced at time of injury. **(B)** demonstrates a similar injury in a paediatric where the fracture of the neck is a Salter-Harris 2 injury through the physeal plate and metaphysis (hollow arrow). (Source: STATdx © Elsevier.)

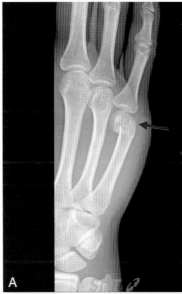

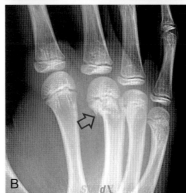

Typical mechanism of injury:
- Punch injury: associate with more of a 'swing' punch than a jab

Clinical presentation:
- Most commonly young men
- Focal pain and swelling over the little finger metacarpal with deformity or loss of the knuckle

Appearance:
- Usually an oblique fracture of the neck of the little (and, less commonly, ring) finger metacarpal
- Sometimes involves the shaft or head but is usually extra-articular
- There is volar (anterior) angulation of the distal part of the fracture, best assessed on the oblique/lateral projections
- Soft tissue swelling adjacent to the injury
- In paediatrics it appears as a Salter-Harris II fracture through the physeal plate and metaphysis

Incidentally metacarpal fractures of trained/professional fighters tend to occur of the longer index and middle (2nd and 3rd) metacarpals, as they tend to strike first.

Open Fracture of the Metacarpal Head

Sometimes referred to as a 'fight bite', these injuries occur when a punch to the mouth results in a tooth causing an open intra-articular fracture to the head of the affected metacarpal. The nature of the injury makes them prone to soft tissue, joint (septic arthritis), and bone infection (osteomyelitis). Sometimes a fragment of a tooth can be seen as a foreign body lodged within the hand, and there is often injury to the overlying extensor tendon to the finger.

Typical mechanism of injury:
- Punch injury to the mouth

Clinical presentation:
- Most commonly young men
- Focal pain and swelling over the MCP joint/metacarpal
- Penetrating injury/soft tissue laceration

Appearance:
- Impacted fracture to head of metacarpal; depression or cortical step
- Soft tissue laceration
- Evaluate for foreign body adjacent to metacarpal head (tooth)

Carpometacarpal Joint Fracture-Dislocations (Fig. 4.60)

There are a range of injuries of the base of the metacarpals and CMC joints that can occur: fractures, dislocations, and fracture-dislocations. Most affect multiple metacarpals, commonly involving the ring and little finger (4th and 5th) metacarpals. These types of injuries are not uncommonly missed due to the complex anatomy of this area.

It is important to assess the bases of the metacarpals for fracture and the spaces between them and the CMC joints for dislocation on both hand and wrist projections (Figs. 4.31, 4.56, and 4.57). It is also important to assess the carpal bones, as associated fractures (particularly to the hamate) can occur.

Dislocations tend to occur with the metacarpals displacing dorsally most typically. CT imaging is commonly used to assess the complexity of injuries

Fig. 4.60 CMC fracture-dislocation; index (2nd) to little (5th) metacarpals and CMC joints. A, DP projection demonstrates overlap between the base of the 2nd to 5th metacarpals (solid lines) and the distal carpals, with resultant loss of the CMC joint spaces, caused by dislocation. A possible fracture fragment is also suggested (hollow arrow). **B,** The oblique projection demonstrates dorsal dislocation of at least one metacarpal in particular (arrow). A fracture fragment is identified (hollow arrow). (Source: STATdx © Elsevier.)

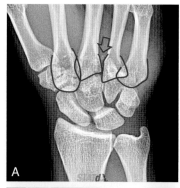

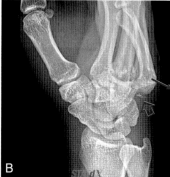

which cannot always be visualised completely on radiographs, particularly small intra-articular fracture fragments.

Typical mechanism of injury:
- Usually high velocity, for example, road traffic collisions, fall from height
- Hyperflexion/hyperextension with rotation

Clinical presentation:
- Focal tenderness, swelling, and deformity

Appearance:
- Dependent on injury; fracture of base of metacarpal(s), dislocation at CMC, or combination. May involve one metacarpal but more commonly multiple
- Cortical step/interruption to base of metacarpal; lucent/sclerotic lines within bone
- DP projection:
    - Widening/loss of spaces between metacarpal bases.
    - Loss of normal CMC joint spaces and 'zigzag' appearance.
    - Overlap of base of metacarpals with distal carpals
    - Possible hamate fracture
- Oblique/lateral projections:
    - Dorsal (normally) dislocation of affected metacarpals
    - Interruption of line following dorsal aspect of metacarpals and carpals.
- Overlying soft tissue swelling.

THUMB

The thumb, like the fingers, consists of several joints and bones which must be examined individually and as a unit.

 INSIGHT

There are a number of common accessory sesamoid bones which may be found in the hand which should not be misinterpreted for avulsion fractures. They should appear smooth and round and will appear adjacent to a joint. The numbers vary from person to person but the most common are found adjacent to the volar aspect of the thumb MCP joint (Figs. 4.56 and 4.61)

Systematic Approach

Radiographic appearances of the thumb (Fig. 4.61)

Anteroposterior/posteroanterior and lateral projections

Follow the standard approach to the AABCSS in addition to:

Adequacy	• AP/PA – is the thumb extended; can we visualise the IP, MCP, and CMC joint? • Lateral – are the condyles of the proximal phalanx superimposed? • Is the thumb clear of superimposition by other bones of the hand?
Alignment	• Does the base of the thumb metacarpal articulate with the trapezium? • Are the bones aligned at the IP and MCP joints?

Bones	• Assess each bone in turn looking for cortical steps/bumps, internal lucent/sclerotic lines, and assess the shape. Follow:
	  • Distal phalanx
	  • Proximal phalanx
	  • Metacarpal
	  • Trapezium
	  • Any other bones included on the projections
	• Remember not to confuse the sesamoid bones with fracture

Cartilage (Joint spaces)	• Assess for widening/narrowing across the whole joint/one aspect of the joint:
	  • IP joint
	  • MCP joint
	  • CMC joint between metacarpal and trapezium
	• Assess for intra-articular fracture, especially of the base of the thumb metacarpal

Soft tissues	• Is there soft tissue swelling, laceration, or air? • Particularly assess the tissues of the tip of the thumb
Significant areas	• Look for evidence of scaphoid fracture • AP/PA – Assess the ulna (medial) aspect of the proximal phalanx for avulsion fracture • Assess the base of the thumb metacarpal for fracture • Ensure you have reviewed all of the bones on the edge of the images

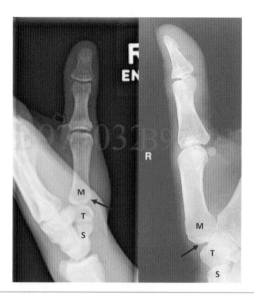

Fig. 4.61 AP and lateral thumb projections: systematic approach. Alignment – does the base of thumb MC (M) articulate with the trapezium (T)? Are the IP and MCP joints aligned? Bones – carefully check ALL of the visible bones: distal phalanx, proximal phalanx, metacarpal (M), trapezium (T); assess all remaining visible bones. Cartilage – any widening/ narrowing of the IP, MCP, and CMC joints? Assess the articular surface of the thumb metacarpal (M) for fracture (arrow). Soft tissues – is there any soft tissue swelling, laceration, or air? Significant areas – scaphoid (S), avulsion fracture ulna aspect of base of proximal phalanx (hollow arrow), base of thumb metacarpal (M), bones on edge of images.

Fractures

Like the hand and fingers, the thumb is prone to injury through a range of mechanisms such as punch and sports injuries. It is also important to consider scaphoid injuries when imaging the thumb, and vice versa, as clinically they can present in a similar way.

Base of Thumb (1st) Metacarpal Fractures (Figs. 4.62 and 4.63)

Occur in three main patterns; the transverse fracture is extra-articular and occurs through the base of the metacarpal, distal to the CMC joint.

The *Bennett fracture* (described by Edward Bennett in 1882) is an oblique intra-articular fracture into the CMC joint, and the Rolando fracture (Silvio Rolando in 1910) is a comminuted intra-articular fracture involving the CMC joint.

With these two types of injury, the smaller volar fragment remains articulating with the trapezium whilst the distal larger part (and rest of thumb) is normally displaced dorsally and proximally due to the pull of adjacent muscles.

Typical mechanism of injury:

- Axial (longitudinal) force on the thumb, typically with it flexed, such as when forming a fist
- Typically the result of punch injuries (particularly if thumb tucked under fingers)

Fig. 4.62 Bennett fracture. Triangular fracture fragment (hollow arrow) remains articulating with the trapezium (T), whilst the remainder of the thumb is displaced proximally and towards the radius (arrow). The fracture is intra-articular, as it involves the thumb CMC joint with the trapezium. (Source: STATdx © Elsevier.)

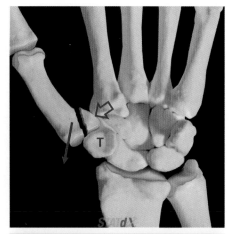

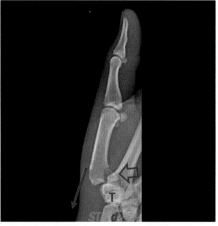

Fig. 4.63 Rolando fracture. Comminuted intra-articular fracture (hollow arrows) of the base of thumb metacarpal with proximal and radial displacement of the thumb (arrow). This example does not have the typical 'T' or 'Y' shape. (Source: STATdx © Elsevier.)

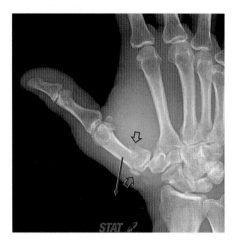

Clinical presentation:
- Focal tenderness over base of thumb/carpals (similar to scaphoid)
- Swelling and deformity

Appearance:
- Transverse fracture:
  - Transverse fracture within base of thumb metacarpal, distal to joint
  - No interruption of articular surface of base of thumb
  - Typically angulated laterally/dorsally away from rest of hand
- Bennett fracture (Fig. 4.62):
  - Oblique fracture within base of thumb metacarpal
  - Involves joint surface of base of thumb into CMC joint with trapezium
  - Smaller triangular fragment volarly (next to index metacarpal) remains *in situ* articulating with trapezium
  - Larger fragment (the thumb metacarpal) is subluxed or dislocated dorsally and proximally towards the radius
- Rolando fracture (Fig. 4.63):
  - Similar to Bennett, but fracture is comminuted; typically either in the shape of a 'T' or a 'Y'.

Skier's Thumb
(Fig. 4.64)

On both the medial (ulna) and lateral (radial) aspects of the MCP and IP joints of the thumb and fingers are a pair of collateral ligaments helping to stabilise the joint. Forced abduction of the thumb at the MCP joint may cause either an avulsion/rupture of the ulna collateral ligament (on the side nearest the rest of the metacarpals) or an avulsion fracture of the base of the proximal phalanx.

Acute ulna collateral ligament avulsion is commonly known as *skier's thumb*, so called by the thumb being forcibly abducted by a ski pole during a fall. A chronic form, known as *gamekeeper's thumb*, is seen as a repetitive strain of the ligament (and not really a fracture). It gets its eponym due to the repetitive actions from dispatching game.

Fig. 4.64 Skier's thumb. An avulsion fracture (arrow) from the base of the ulna aspect of the base of the proximal phalanx of the thumb. This is the site of insertion of the ulna collateral ligament. This is a relatively large fragment, they can be more subtle, and there is no joint space widening which is also often demonstrated. (Source: STATdx © Elsevier.)

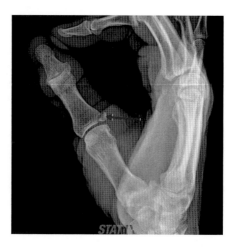

Typical mechanism of injury:
- Acute; forced hyperabduction (away from rest of hand) at the MCP joint.
- Typically as a result of falls but specifically in skiing injuries

Clinical presentation:
- Focal pain and swelling
- Instability (laxity) of the thumb MCP joint

Appearance:
- AP/PA projection: avulsion fracture base of proximal phalanx, ulna aspect (closest to other metacarpals). Will not be evident if ligament avulsion/tear only
- AP/PA projection: widening of ulna aspect of MCP joint, angulation of phalanges towards radial side
- Soft tissue swelling over MCP joint

 INSIGHT

Sometimes describing the medial/lateral relationship in the hand can be confusing. Remember that anatomical locations/descriptions always revert back to the normal anatomical position with the hands facing anteriorly down by your side. The medial aspect is closer to the body on the ulna side of the forearm/wrist. The lateral aspect is away from the body on the radial side of the forerarm/wrist.

FINGERS

Adequacy

Adequate positioning of the finger, particularly on the lateral projection, is essential to ensure the subtlest of injuries are likely to be observed. It is essential to try and ensure the phalanges are not superimposed by other structures (such as the other fingers or dressings), the fingers are extended (where the injury allows) to visualise the joint spaces, and the condyles of the phalanges are superimposed on the lateral projection.

Of course, this is dependent on the patient's symptoms but should be considered when positioning and interpreting the radiographs.

If imaging multiple fingers, it may be necessary to obtain separate images of each digit, particularly on the lateral projection.

 INSIGHT

A true lateral is essential to fully assess finger injuries. Pads are often used to help extend the affected digit and prevent the superimposition of other structures. They should be used with caution, however, as they can reduce fractures and joint space widening, thereby obscuring or hiding subtle injuries.

Alignment

Assess the alignment and shape of the entire digit. Certain injuries (e.g. hyper-flexion or extension) can cause injuries which alter the position of the respective phalanges from their normal alignment when the fingers are extended. Sub-optimal positioning can also mimic misalignment.

Bones

The distal phalanges and tufts are prone to crush injuries and so should be assessed carefully.

In understanding where injuries occur (and where to look) it is perhaps important to remember the anatomy of the flexor and extensor muscles/tendons (Figs. 4.67 and 4.68) of the fingers, as these are common sites of injury:

- The extensor digitorum muscles (on the dorsal aspect) extend the digit. The main insertion is at the dorsal aspect of the base of the distal phalanx. This results in us only being able to extend our digit as a whole.
- The flexor digitorum muscles (on the volar aspect) flex the digit. The main insertions are at the volar surface at the base of the distal phalanx and on the shaft of the middle phalanx. This allows us to flex our fingers at both the distal and proximal interphalangeal joints independently.
- The volar aspect of the PIP joint of the fingers has a thickening of the fibrous joint capsule called the volar plate (Fig. 4.68). Both this and other joint ligaments insert at the base of the middle phalanx.

As a result of this anatomy, it is important to carefully assess the bases of the dorsal surface of the distal phalanx and volar surfaces of the distal and middle phalanges for fracture.

Cartilage

Assess each joint for joint space for widening/narrowing either the entire joint or one side of the joint.

Look carefully within the joint for small bone fragments.

Soft Tissues

Check for general soft tissue swelling on each projection. If there is soft tissue swelling, assess the adjacent area of bone/joint.

Foreign bodies are also fairly common in the fingers, especially with soft tissue lacerations, which may be caused by crush and other types of injuries.

Look for the presence of air within the soft tissues, especially where fractures are present (in particular the end of the digits). Involvement of the nail bed is also usually indicative of an open fracture.

Significant Areas

As indicated above, specific areas to check are bases of the dorsal aspect of the distal phalanges and the volar aspect of the distal and proximal phalanges, as well as within their adjacent joint spaces.

Ensure you have assessed each bone individually, including those on the edge of the images (such as the head of metacarpal and adjacent fingers) or where superimposed by other anatomy.

Systematic Approach

Radiographic appearances of the finger (Fig. 4.65)

Dorsipalmar and lateral projections

Follow the standard approach to the AABCSS in addition to:

Adequacy	• Ensure digit is not superimposed by other structures (including dressings). • Digits should be extended and joint spaces visualised • Ensure condyles of phalanges are superimposed (lateral projection)
Alignment	• Assess alignment of DIP, PIP, and MCP joints (both projections)

Bones	• Assess each bone in turn looking for cortical steps/bumps, internal lucent/sclerotic lines, and assess the shape. Follow:
	   • Distal phalanx
	   • Middle phalanx
	   • Proximal phalanx
	   • Metacarpal
	   • Any other bones included on the projections
	 • Specifically look for avulsion fractures (lateral projection):
	 • Dorsal aspect base of distal phalanx
	 • Volar aspect base of distal phalanx
	 • Volar aspect base of middle phalanx (volar plate)

Cartilage (Joint spaces)	• Assess for widening/narrowing across the whole joint/one aspect of the joint:
	   • DIP joint
	   • PIP
	   • MCP joint
	 • Assess joint spaces for small intra-articular fragments

Soft tissues	• Is there soft tissue swelling, laceration, or air? • Particularly assess the tissues of the tip of the fingers and nail beds

Significant areas	• Look for subtle avulsion fractures:
	   • Dorsal aspect base of distal phalanx
	   • Volar aspect base of distal phalanx
	   • Volar aspect base of middle phalanx (volar plate)
	   • Within DIP and PIP joints
	 • Ensure you have reviewed all of the bones on the edge of the images

Fractures/Trauma

Injuries to bones, joints, and soft tissues are extremely common. They are also extremely important, since delayed diagnosis or management can lead to loss

Mallet Finger (Fig. 4.67) Caused by an avulsion of the insertion of the extensor digitorum tendon on the dorsal surface of the base of the distal phalanx. Avulsion of a small bone fragment, tendon avulsion, or tendon rupture may all occur. Be aware that use of pads to position the finger (and reduce deformity) may obscure all imaging appearances of this injury.

Typical mechanism of injury:
- Forced flexion of DIP joint, for example, stubbing finger or ball striking end of finger

Clinical presentation:
- Patient unable to extend finger
- Fixed '*mallet*' flexion deformity at the DIP joint

Appearance:
- Best visualised on lateral projection
- Volar angulation (flexion) at DIP joint. Articular surfaces still opposing (not dislocated)
- Small avulsion/triangular fracture fragment from dorsal surface of base of distal phalanx (may not be present if soft tissue injury only)
- Soft tissue swelling over dorsal aspect of the joint.

Fig. 4.67 Mallet finger. The extensor digitorum tendon (hollow arrow) inserts at the base of the dorsal aspect of the distal phalanx and helps extend the digit. Avulsion of either the tendon or a bone fracture fragment (arrows) results in flexion at the DIP joint (curved arrows). Note the location of the flexor tendons on the volar aspect of the finger and their insertion on the base of the middle and distal phalanges (*). (Source: STATdx © Elsevier.)

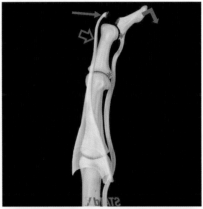
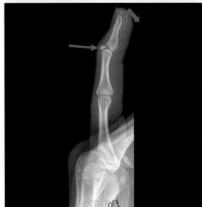

Volar Plate Avulsion Fracture (Fig. 4.68)

The volar plate is prone to avulsion injuries either to the plate itself (not visible on radiographs) or to the base of the proximal phalanx.

A similar avulsion can also be seen at the volar surface of the base of the distal phalanx at the insertion of the flexor digitorum tendon (there is no volar plate of the DIP joint). This is called the 'rugger jersey finger' caused by grabbing the clothing of an opponent.

Fractures associated with these injuries can be extremely small and subtle; a true lateral projection gives the best opportunity to visualise them. The use of pads to position the finger can also cause them to be missed.

Typical mechanism of injury:
- Hyperextension, for example, catching a ball
- Forced extension, for example, when holding onto an item of clothing such as a rugby shirt

Clinical presentation:
- Focal pain, bruising, and swelling
- Difficulty flexing joint

Appearance:
- Best visualised on lateral projection
- Triangular or very fine bone fragment adjacent to volar aspect of base of middle phalanx (volar plate) or distal phalanx
- Soft tissue swelling

Fig. 4.68 Volar plate avulsion fracture. (A), Occur at the base of middle phalanx where the volar plate inserts (hollow arrow). Hyperextension injury may cause a soft tissue or bony avulsion fracture at this point (arrows). Bony avulsions can be large **(B)** or very small **(C),** which is why a well-positioned lateral projection is essential. (Source: STATdx © Elsevier.)

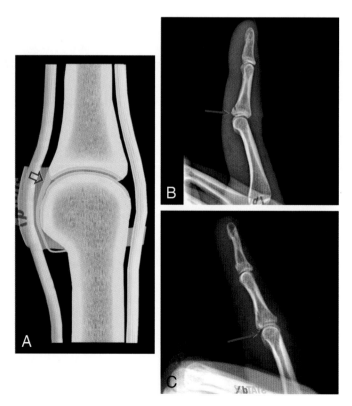

Crush Fractures/ Amputations (Fig. 4.69)

These can range from simple crush injuries causing comminuted fractures to the distal phalangeal tufts, open fractures involving the nail bed or soft tissue lacerations, and complete amputations to digits.

It is important when assessing such injuries to consider the degree of comminution (i.e. the number of fragments) and that there may be a communication with the air (i.e. an open fracture) and a higher risk of infection, for example, soft tissue lacerations, damage to the nail, and air within the soft tissues. Dressings can obscure/mimic fractures and soft tissue injuries.

Salter-Harris II Fractures (Fig. 4.70)

As with other paediatric injuries, the physeal (growth) plates of the digits are prone to injury, particularly at the bases of the proximal phalanges. Whilst other types of fracture can occur (particularly Salter-Harris I and III), most common are Salter-Harris II injuries, which involve a fracture of the physeal plate and metaphysis distal to the plate.

These can be subtle but commonly are displaced with angulation and mistaken for dislocations (though the joint is intact).

Typical mechanism of injury:
- Variable; as per other fractures and dislocations
- Hyperextension/flexion, direct blows

Fig. 4.69 Crush injuries/ amputations. A, – Crush injury of the thumb resulting in an oblique fracture of the distal phalangeal tuft. Air and laceration of the soft tissues (arrows) indicate this is an open fracture, probably involving the nail. **B,** Traumatic amputation of the index and middle fingers. (Source: STATdx © Elsevier.)

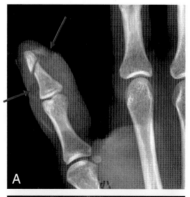

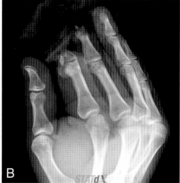

Fig. 4.70 Salter-Harris II fractures. Most common on the radial side of the proximal phalanges, the fracture extends through the physeal plate, which is not always visible if undisplaced (hollow arrow), and metaphysis (arrows). **A,** PA projection of the right thumb; fracture of the proximal phalanx with displacement. **B,** AP oblique of the left hand; fractures of the ring and little (more subtle) finger proximal phalanges. (Source: STATdx © Elsevier.)

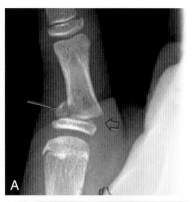

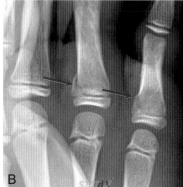

Clinical presentation:
- Paediatrics/young adolescents; until fusion of physeal plates
- Most commonly of proximal phalanx of ring and little fingers
- Focal pain, deformity, soft tissue swelling

Appearance:
- Dependent on severity/displacement
- Widening of physeal plate (not always visible)
- Oblique fracture or buckling of cortex of metaphysis, distal to physeal plate
- Angulation of distal part (rest of finger) towards fracture fragment

 INSIGHT

It is worth remembering the normal developmental anatomy of the hand. In immature paediatric skeletons, normally:
- the metacarpals of the fingers have an epiphysis and physeal plate at the head but not the base
- the thumb metacarpal has an epiphysis and physeal plate at its base but not its head
- the phalanges of the thumb and fingers have an epiphysis and physeal plate at their base but not their head

SHOULDER GIRDLE   5

In this chapter we will consider the interpretation of skeletal radiographs of the shoulder girdle, which consists of the humerus, clavicle, and scapula bones as well as the glenohumeral, acromioclavicular, and sternoclavicular joints.

For many, the shoulder is a complex and daunting area to interpret, so in order to do this we will break down into the main projections undertaken and consider them individually. It may be worth revisiting the anatomy of the shoulder girdle before progressing with this chapter.

ANTEROPOSTERIOR PROJECTION

The AP projection provides an overview of the structures of the shoulder girdle, including the proximal humerus, scapula, clavicle, and glenohumeral and acromioclavicular joints. Since the AP projection provides visualisation of the entire shoulder girdle, because of the nature and complexity of the anatomy, it does not necessarily provide a thorough assessment of all structures.

There is a lot to review, so our systematic approach is required to break it down into manageable pieces.

Adequacy

When positioning, the scapula should be in contact with the detector so that this structure is demonstrated en-face and the clavicle is elongated and not foreshortened. Rotation of the patient towards the affected side produces a clearer visualisation of the glenohumeral joint space but in turn distorts other structures.

In order to provide visualisation of the humeral head, and greater tuberosity in particular, the arm should be slightly abducted and externally rotated so that the greater tuberosity is in profile. Internal rotation of the humerus brings the greater tuberosity to be superimposed and the humeral head appears more rounded.

Ensure that the entire clavicle (particularly medial end) and scapula (particularly inferior angle) are included on the image.

Fig 5.1 AP shoulder projection: alignment.
Does the smooth humeral head (solid curved line) articulate with glenoid fossa (round circle)? AC joint; do the inferior surfaces of the acromion (A) and distal clavicle (C) follow a smooth line (dotted line)? Does the medial end of the clavicle (M) articulate with the sternum (S)? (Source: Bontrager's Textbook of Radiographic Positioning and Related Anatomy, Tenth Edition, 2021.)

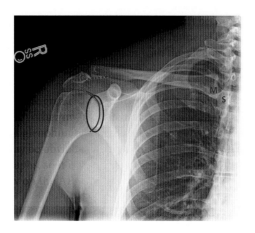

◉ INSIGHT

When the arm is externally rotated, the humeral head appears more like a hockey stick in shape, and the greater tuberosity is visualised. When internally rotated, it becomes more rounded, like a lightbulb, which can mimic pathology (particularly a posterior dislocation). The greater tuberosity is no longer visualised, since it is superimposed on the humeral head, so fractures here are not visible (see Fig. 5.16).

Alignment (Fig. 5.1)

Ensure the rounded articular surface of the humeral head is in contact with the glenoid fossa. The proximal end of the clavicle should also align with the sternum.

Normal alignment of the acromioclavicular (AC) joint can be ascertained by drawing a line along the inferior aspect of the acromion process, which should then follow along the inferior aspect of the distal clavicle. Any steps in this line (alongside the normal distances discussed below) suggest injury to the AC joint.

Bones (Figs. 5.2 and 5.3)

The bone's external cortex and internal texture should be carefully assessed by looking at the proximal humerus, clavicle, and scapula in turn. Specific care should be taken to look at the midshaft of the clavicle, since fractures here may be undisplaced and superimposed by the ribs.

The greater tuberosity and lateral aspect of the humeral head are common fracture sites and so should be smooth and without depression.

The surgical neck of humerus is also a common fracture site though usually obvious.

Fig 5.2 AP shoulder projection: bones (1).
Assess the: humerus (H), especially the shape of the greater tuberosity (T) and humeral head (solid line); scapula (dotted line); clavicle (C). (Source: Bontrager's Textbook of Radiographic Positioning and Related Anatomy, Tenth Edition, 2021.)

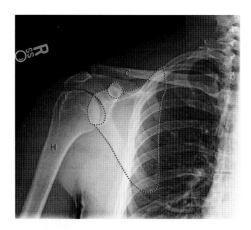

Fig 5.3 AP shoulder projection: bones (2).
Assess the: mid clavicle (arrow) for subtle fractures; surgical neck of humerus (dotted line); ribs (1–9). Look for small avulsion fractures adjacent to inferior glenoid (arrowhead). (Source: Bontrager's Textbook of Radiographic Positioning and Related Anatomy, Tenth Edition, 2021.)

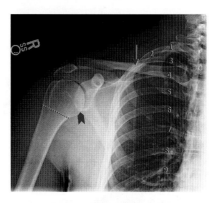

 INSIGHT

In paediatrics the physeal growth plate may be mistaken for fracture. It lies more proximal than the surgical neck (where many fractures occur), appears less well defined and lucent than a fracture, and is normally curved or 'V' shaped. As the orientation of the physeal plate is not always parallel with the X-ray beam, it may appear as two separate lines (Fig. 5.4).

Similarly, the AC joint may also appear abnormally widened until the acromion has ossified.

Also remember to assess each rib in turn. Start medially from the first rib where it joins the spine and follow it laterally to its anterior end on the sternum. Then move to the second and so on.

Cartilage (Fig. 5.5)

Assessment of a number of joint spaces and measurements should be made.
Glenohumeral joint space:
An AP projection will not provide clear visualisation of the glenohumeral joint space, since the glenoid and joint is not parallel to the X-ray beam (it lies

Fig 5.4 AP Shoulder projection: paediatric shoulder. Note the normal shape and appearance of the paediatric physeal plate (solid line). Sometimes a second line, though not in this case (but illustrated by dotted line), may be demonstrated depending on the relationship between the angle of the X-ray beam and the physeal plate. Lack of ossification of the acromion makes the AC joint appear widened when it is not (arrow). (Source: STATdx © Elsevier.)

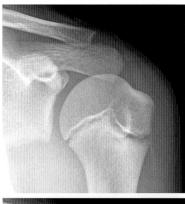

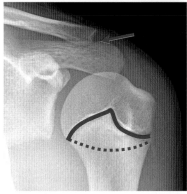

Fig 5.5 AP shoulder projection: cartilage (joints). Glenohumeral joint space: head of humerus and glenoid fossa (solid lines) overlapping with no clear joint space. Acromioclavicular joint space (arrow): not widened (max ~8 mm). Coracoclavicular distance (curved arrow): space between coracoid process (C) and conoid tubercle (T); not widened (max ~12 mm). Subacromial space (arrowhead): between inferior aspect acromion (A) and humeral head (H); not widened (max ~15 mm). (Source: Bontrager's Textbook of Radiographic Positioning and Related Anatomy, Tenth Edition, 2021.)

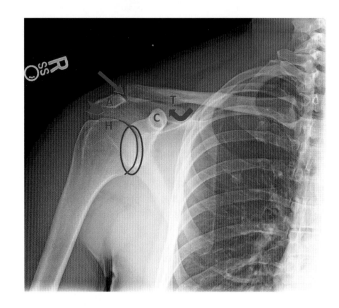

approximately 30° from the sagittal plane) and therefore cannot be accurately assessed (Fig. 5.7). There should, however, be a small amount of some overlap/superimposition of the humeral head on the glenoid fossa, without a space seen between them (unless the patient is turned towards the affected side).

AC joint space:

It should measure up to approximately 8 mm (dependent on patient size), so assess this for widening, which may indicate disruption.

Coracoclavicular distance:

The space between the conoid process on the inferior aspect of the clavicle and the coracoid process should measure up to approximately 12 mm in size (again dependent on patient size). Widening of this distance alongside widening of the AC joint space suggests injury.

Sub-acromial space:

The distance between the inferior aspect of the acromion and superior aspect of the humeral head varies (both by patient and with positioning) but is typically up to approximately 15 mm. It should be assessed for an increase in this distance, which may be a result of glenohumeral joint subluxation/dislocation or other soft tissue injury (such as rupture of the rotator cuff tendons).

 INSIGHT

Degenerative changes to the AC joint and rotator cuff tendons often cause the AC joint and sub-acromial space to narrow, particularly in the elderly or with previous injury.

Soft Tissues (Fig. 5.6)

Assess for soft tissue swelling, particularly around the proximal humerus and AC joint.

Occasionally injury may cause a large effusion, or *lipohaemarthrosis* (see Chapter 6, page 158), in the sub-acromial space, which subluxes the humeral head inferiorly from its normal articulation with the glenoid fossa. An effusion will appear as a soft tissue density and is suggestive of injury (bone or soft tissue) whilst the double density and horizontal line of a lipohaemarthrosis indicates the presence of an intra-articular fracture.

Whilst not a chest X-ray, it is important to assess the chest for underlying trauma/pathology. It is outside the scope of this book to consider chest interpretation, but some key things to consider when looking at the chest include:

- Whether the lung markings come to the periphery of the chest wall.
- Whether the edge of a lung can be seen (particularly in the apex). Both of these signs may indicate a pneumothorax.
- Focal masses or areas of increased opacity in the visualised lung.

Any such appearances may warrant further imaging of the chest.

Fig 5.6 AP shoulder projection: soft tissues. Any soft tissue swelling, particularly over upper arm and AC joint? Any evidence of effusion/ lipohaemarthrosis in subacromial space (arrow) and depressing humerus? Lung markings extending to chest wall (arrowhead). Any evidence of a lung edge, particularly in the apex (curved arrow)? Any focal lung opacities? (Source: Bontrager's Textbook of Radiographic Positioning and Related Anatomy, Tenth Edition, 2021.)

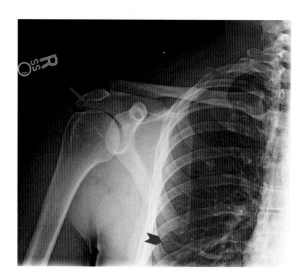

⊙ INSIGHT

The presence of rib or scapula fractures increases the likelihood of lung pathology. Fractures to the first rib and scapula in particular require significant trauma, which may also cause associated lung or mediastinal injury.

Significant Areas

As always, the systematic approach should hopefully have identified any potential injuries; however, there are a number of areas of the AP shoulder where subtle injuries are found or pathology missed.

- The greater tuberosity for small avulsion fractures or concavity of its surface due to compression injuries
- The inferior aspect of the glenoid rim; small fractures can occur here
- The scapula, ribs, and chest; look for subtle fractures

Systematic Approach

Radiographic appearances of the shoulder girdle, AP projection (Figs. 5.1–5.6)

Anteroposterior projection
Follow the standard approach to the AABCSS in addition to:

Adequacy	• Ensure the clavicle and scapula are not foreshortened and are fully visualised
	• Is the arm externally rotated; is the greater tuberosity in profile?
Alignment	• Does the smooth round articular surface of the humeral head articulate with the glenoid fossa?
	• AC joint – inferior surfaces of acromion and distal clavicle along same line; any steps/ interruptions?
	• Does the medial end of the clavicle articulate with the sternum?

Bones	• Follow the cortex and assess the internal structure of the humerus, clavicle, and scapula in turn
	• Look for subtle fractures in the mid-clavicle where superimposed by the ribs
	• Assess the greater tuberosity and shape of the lateral head of humerus for any depression/concavity
	• Look for surgical neck fracture
	• Ribs – start at 1st rib and move inferiorly; follow from vertebra and round to anterior aspect
Cartilage (Joint spaces)	• Glenohumeral joint – are the humeral head and glenoid fossa overlapping?
	• AC joint space – is it widened (~8 mm maximum)?
	• Coracoclavicular distance – is it widened (~12 mm maximum)?
	• Sub-acromial space – is it widened (~15 mm maximum), is the humeral head depressed from the glenoid fossa?
Soft tissues	• Any evidence of soft tissue swelling?
	• Evidence of effusion/lipohaemarthrosis in the sub-acromial space?
	• Assess the visible chest:
	• Do the lung markings reach the chest wall?
	• Is there a visible lung edge – particularly in the apex?
	• Any evidence of increased opacity in the lung?
Significant areas	• Assess the greater tuberosity – any avulsion fractures or concavity of the surface?
	• Any fractures of the ribs or scapula?
	• Review the visible chest
	• Inferior glenoid rim – any fracture fragments?

AXIAL (OR MODIFIED AXIAL) PROJECTION

A secondary projection of the shoulder is always required with a history of trauma; commonly, this is either the axial or modified axial projection. The main aim of the secondary projection is to confirm the presence and direction of a glenohumeral joint dislocation, though it can also be used to identify additional injuries not seen on the AP.

One thing to consider when assessing the integrity of the glenohumeral joint is that only approximately one-third of the articular surface of the humeral head articulates with the glenoid fossa at any one time.

 INSIGHT

These projections are often confusing to review (or even looked at upside down) because anatomy is not understood. One tip is to remember that all of the projections of the scapula (coracoid, glenoid, and acromion) point anteriorly (Fig. 5.7).

Systematic Approach

Radiographic appearances of the shoulder girdle, axial (or modified axial) projection (Figs. 5.7 and 5.8)

Axial/modified axial projection

Follow the standard approach to the AABCSS in addition to:

Adequacy	• Ensure the glenoid fossa and humeral head are clearly visualised
Alignment	• Does the smooth round articular surface of the humeral head articulate with the glenoid fossa? • Does the distal clavicle articulate with the acromion process?

Bones	• Follow the cortex and assess the internal structure of the humerus, clavicle, and scapula in turn
	• Look for fractures of:
	  • Coracoid process
	  • Acromion process
	  • Glenoid rim
	  • Spine of scapula
	  • Surgical neck of humerus
	• Assess the smooth articular surface of the humeral head for depressions

Cartilage (Joint spaces)	• Glenohumeral joint – is there a clear joint space?
Soft tissues	• Any evidence of soft tissue swelling?
Significant areas	• Look for small avulsion fractures related to the glenoid rim

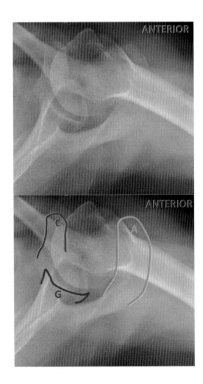

Fig 5.7 Axial (right) shoulder projection: anatomy. Remember, all processes of the scapula point anteriorly. Coracoid process (C – red); glenoid (G – blue); acromion (A – green). This image also demonstrates the normal alignment of the glenohumeral joint and why a clear joint space is not visualised on the AP projection. (Source: Rockwood and Matsen's The Shoulder, Sixth Edition, 2022.)

Fig 5.8 Axial (right) shoulder projection: systematic approach. Alignment – articular surface of humeral head (H) with glenoid fossa (G); distal clavicle (C) with acromion (A). Bones – assess clavicle, humerus, and scapula in turn; humeral head (H) for depressions in cortex; assess for fractures of: coracoid process (CP), acromion (A), glenoid (G), spine of scapula (S), surgical neck of humerus (dotted line). Cartilage – glenohumeral joint (between H and G); clear joint space. Soft tissues – is there any soft tissue swelling? Significant areas – avulsion fractures adjacent to glenoid rim (G). (Source: Rockwood and Matsen's The Shoulder, Sixth Edition, 2022.)

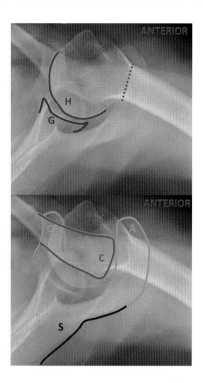

⊙ INSIGHT

Each process of the scapula has its own ossification centre which is evident in paediatrics. In adults it is possible to fracture these. In some adults, though, these ossification centres do not unite and remain visible as normal variants (Fig. 5.9)

Y-VIEW (OR LATERAL SCAPULA) PROJECTION

Like the axial projection, the anatomy on this projection may cause some confusion. Essentially the 'Y' is formed by the:

- coracoid process anteriorly,
- the acromion process posteriorly, and
- the body of the scapula inferiorly.

The junction of the 'Y' is the location of the glenoid fossa, and so the head of humerus should also articulate with this in the middle of the 'Y'. The ribs lie anterior to the scapula.

The main role of this projection secondary to the AP is to assess for dislocation of the glenohumeral joint and displacement of proximal humeral fractures but also to assess the scapula for fracture.

Fig 5.9 Normal ossification centres. A, The normal paediatric epiphyses of the humeral head (H), acromion (A), glenoid (G), and coracoid process should not be mistaken for fractures. As described in Fig. 5.4, the physeal plate of the humerus can demonstrate two separate lines (arrows). **B,** Os acromiale. In this mature skeleton, a residual ossification centre of the acromion remains (A) separate from the scapula spine (S) with a gap between them (arrow). It is smooth, round, and corticated, differentiating it from an acromion fracture. (Source: Diagnostic Imaging: Musculoskeletal, STATdx © Elsevier.)

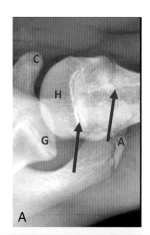

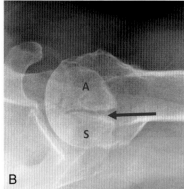

Systematic Approach

Radiographic appearances of the shoulder girdle, Y-view/lateral scapula projection (Fig. 5.10)

Y-view/lateral scapula projection
Follow the standard approach to the AABCSS in addition to:

Adequacy	• Ensure the scapula is clear from the rib cage • Is the inferior angle of the scapula included on the image?
Alignment	• Does the head of humerus lie within the three points of the 'Y' (within the glenoid fossa)? • Is there overlap between the distal clavicle and acromion (the AC joint)?

Bones	• Follow the cortex and assess the internal structure of the humerus and scapula in turn
	• Look for fractures of the other bones included on the image:
	  • Clavicle
	  • Ribs

Cartilage (Joint spaces)	• There are not any joint spaces that can be assessed

Fig 5.10 Y-view/lateral scapula projection (A).
B, The "Y" is formed at the junction of the acromion (A), coracoid (C), and body of scapula (S). **C,** The glenoid fossa is where the points of the Y meet (though not visible) **D,** The humeral head (H) should lie within the points of the Y in the glenoid fossa (arrow). The ribs lie anterior to the scapula. (Source: From Lampignano, Bontrager's Textbook of Radiographic Positioning and Related Anatomy, 10e, Elsevier)

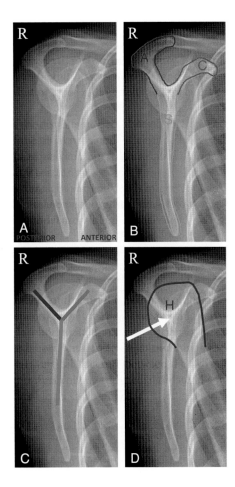

| Soft tissues | • Any evidence of soft tissue swelling? Assess those posterior to the scapula in particular |

Soft tissues
- Any evidence of soft tissue swelling? Assess those posterior to the scapula in particular
- Assess the visible chest:
  - Do the lung markings reach the chest wall?
  - Is there a visible lung edge – particularly in the apex?
  - Any evidence of increased opacity in the lung?

Significant areas
- Assess for fractures of the acromion and coracoid processes
- Look for subtle fractures of the body of the scapula

Fractures/Trauma

Injuries to the shoulder girdle are common and may be a combination of fracture, dislocation/subluxation, and soft tissue injury (many of which are not visible on radiographs). The main types of injury that may occur and that are covered in this chapter are:
- Glenohumeral dislocations (anterior/posterior/inferior) and associated fractures
- Greater tuberosity fractures

- Proximal humeral fractures
- Scapula fractures; body, coracoid, and acromion
- Acromioclavicular (AC) joint subluxation/dislocation
- Sternoclavicular (SC) joint subluxation/dislocation
- Clavicle fractures (covered later in the chapter, on page 146)

Glenohumeral Joint Dislocations

Dislocations of the head of humerus from the glenoid fossa are the most commonly dislocations in the body (up to 50%).

The complexity of these dislocations, and their accompanying injuries, deserves some more detailed consideration.

 INSIGHT

The force of the injury (and during subsequent reduction) and the strength of the supporting muscles which act on the humeral head often mean there are associated fractures to the head of humerus and glenoid rim. Many dislocations may relocate spontaneously (especially in recurrent injuries), so it is important to review shoulder images for these following a history of trauma.

Anterior Glenohumeral Joint Dislocation

(Figs. 5.11–5.13)

Over 95% of glenohumeral dislocations are anterior, making it the most common dislocation in the body. The humeral head normally displaces anteriorly, inferiorly, and medially from the glenoid fossa so that it lies inferiorly to the coracoid process.

Displacement of the humerus causes it to impact on the inferior aspect of the glenoid rim, which can sometimes also result in:

- An avulsion fracture of the greater tuberosity
- *Hills-Sachs fracture* (or *hatchet deformity*); impaction fracture of the posterosuperior aspect of the head of humerus caused by the glenoid rim
- *Bankart fracture*; bony fracture of the inferior aspect of the glenoid caused by the head of humerus
- *Bankart lesion*; tear of the cartilage labrum of the inferior glenoid (not visible on radiographs)
- Tear of the rotator cuff tendons which support the head of humerus in the glenoid fossa (not directly visible on radiographs)

Whilst the dislocation is usually obvious, these associated injuries are often very subtle (and may require additional imaging such as MRI or ultrasound) and may occur either at the time of the injury or as it is reduced (either spontaneously or in the ED).

Anterior dislocations commonly recur many times (sometimes spontaneously), particularly if they first occur in the young (up to 90% recur). Injury to the supporting soft tissue results in a weakness in them, so the joint dislocates more easily in the future. The associated injuries listed above most commonly occur during the initial dislocation rather than the subsequent ones.

Fig 5.11 Anterior dislocation glenohumeral joint. A, AP projection: the humeral head (H) has displaced inferiorly and medially (arrow) from the glenoid fossa (G) and now lies inferior to the coracoid process (C). **B,** Axial projection: the humeral head (H) has displaced anteriorly (arrow) from the glenoid fossa (G). Note that there are no visible associated injuries on this example. (Source: Diagnostic Imaging: Musculoskeletal, STATdx © Elsevier.)

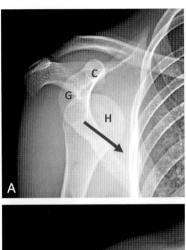

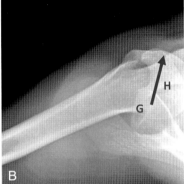

Typical mechanisms of injury:
- Forced abduction/direct blow with arm in abduction and external rotation, for example, fall onto arm held away from body
- Direct blow to posterior aspect shoulder
- Forced traction, 'pulling' humerus out of joint
- Spontaneous following recurrent dislocations

Clinical presentation:
- Severe pain
- Depression inferior to acromion/swelling anteriorly due to displaced head of humerus
- Patient describes shoulder 'popping out'
- Most common in younger adults; recurrence more common in younger patients too
- Hills-Sachs/Bankart fracture or lesion; young adults
- Greater tuberosity fracture/rotator cuff tear; older adults

Radiographic appearance:
- AP projection:
  - Humeral head not overlapping glenoid fossa; lies inferior and medial (often inferior to coracoid process). May be the only finding.

Fig 5.12 Hill-Sachs and Bankart fractures. Post-reduction images (of different patients). **A,** Hills-Sachs fracture; the humerus is now relocated in the glenoid fossa, demonstrating the normal overlap. Note the concavity of the lateral aspect of the head of humerus (arrow) compared to normal (Fig. 5.2), which represents the impaction fracture. **B,** Bankart fracture; the humerus is now relocated in the glenoid fossa. A small fracture fragment of the anterior glenoid is evident (arrow). The axial CT **(C)** of the same patient demonstrates the fracture clearly (arrow). (Source: Diagnostic Imaging: Musculoskeletal, STATdx © Elsevier.)

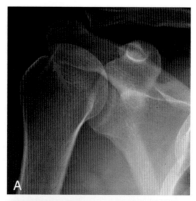

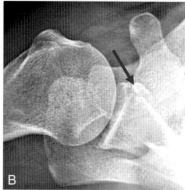

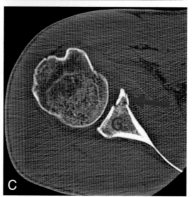

- Hills-Sachs fracture (if present); depression/concavity of superolateral aspect of the head of humerus. Best demonstrated on internal rotation of humerus
- Bankart fracture (if present); small avulsion fracture inferior to glenoid rim
- Axial/modified axial projection:
  - Head of humerus displaced anterior to glenoid fossa
  - Hills-Sachs fracture (if present); depression/concavity of posterior aspect

Fig 5.13 Anterior glenohumeral fracture-dislocation. There is inferomedial displacement of the humeral head (arrow) typical of an anterior dislocation, though it needs confirming on a second projection. There is an associated comminuted fracture of the greater tuberosity (arrowhead). (Source: Diagnostic Imaging: Musculoskeletal, STATdx © Elsevier.)

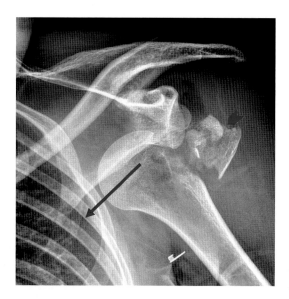

- Bankart fracture (if present); small avulsion fracture anterior to glenoid rim or flattened glenoid rim
  - Y-view/lateral scapula projection:
    - Head of humerus no longer in middle of 'Y'; lying over ribs/inferior to coracoid process
  - Post-reduction imaging:
    - Head of humerus articulating with glenoid fossa (may appear slightly inferior due to soft tissue injury)
    - Appearance of Hills-Sachs/Bankart fractures as described above

Posterior Glenohumeral Joint Dislocation

(Fig. 5.14)

In comparison to anterior dislocations, posterior ones are rare, contributing to less than 5% of glenohumeral dislocations, but often more difficult to identify on imaging, especially on the AP projection, and may be overlooked initially.

The head of humerus displaces posterior to the rim of the glenoid (or may get perched upon it), causing forced internal rotation of the arm. The head of humerus appears more rounded: the '*lightbulb sign*'. This displacement causes apparent widening of the joint space and loss of the normal overlap of the humerus and glenoid fossa on the AP projection.

A vertically orientated impaction fracture (similar to the Hills-Sachs) may often be seen where the anterior head of humerus impacts on the posterior aspect of the glenoid: the '*Trough*' or '*reverse Hills-Sachs*' sign.

It may also cause a fracture to the posterior glenoid rim or cartilage labrum (reverse Bankart fracture/lesion)

Typical mechanisms of injury:

- Strong involuntary muscular movements, for example, epileptic seizure or electric shock
- Less commonly as a result of trauma; may occur due to violent force to anterior aspect of shoulder with arm in internal rotation, or FOOSH (rarely)

Fig 5.14 Posterior glenohumeral joint dislocation. A, AP projection; note the rounded (lightbulb) appearance of the humeral head (compared to Fig. 5.2). There is apparent widening of the glenohumeral joint (*) with loss of the normal overlap between the head of humerus and glenoid fossa. A subtle vertical line (arrowhead) represents an impacted fracture (Trough sign/Reverse Hills-Sachs). **B,** Axial projection (same patient); there is posterior displacement (arrow) of the articular surface of the humeral head (H), which is now perched on the posterior rim of the glenoid (G). The impacted reverse Hill-Sachs fracture is clearly demonstrated of the anteromedial aspect of the humerus (arrowhead). (Source: Diagnostic Imaging: Musculoskeletal, STATdx © Elsevier.)

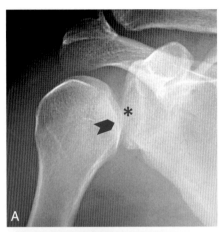

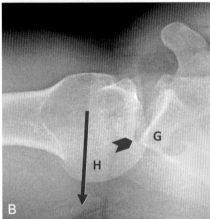

Clinical presentation:
- Pain and limited range of movement
- Flattened anterior shoulder, unable to palpate head of humerus
- More common in older adults (opposite to anterior)

Radiographic appearance:
- AP projection:
  - Lightbulb sign; head of humerus rounded, loss of great tuberosity outline (may be mimicked if arm in internal rotation due to positioning; see Fig. 5.16)
  - Glenohumeral joint space may appear widened; loss of overlap between head of humerus and glenoid fossa
  - Trough sign; vertically orientated sclerotic line due to impacted fracture (if present)
- Axial/modified axial projection:
  - Head of humerus displaced posterior to glenoid fossa; may be perched on posterior glenoid rim

- Trough sign (if present); depression/concavity of anteromedial aspect of head of humerus
- Reverse Bankart fracture (if present); small avulsion fracture to posterior glenoid rim
- Y-view/lateral scapula projection:
  - Head of humerus no longer in the middle of 'Y'; posterior to ribs (towards skin surface)

Inferior Glenohumeral Joint Dislocation (Fig. 5.15)

Rare (less than 1%) form of glenohumeral joint dislocation where the humeral head displaces inferiorly and causes the arm to be abducted above the head (like the patient has their arm up), called *luxatio erecta.*

It may be associated with other injuries including fracture to all bones of the shoulder girdle, rupture of the joint capsule and rotator cuff, and neurovascular injury to the axillary artery and brachial plexus, which may necessitate urgent reduction. It may also be an open injury in the most severe cases.

Typical mechanism of injury:
- Fall onto arm held in full abduction above head; for example, diving injury hitting the bottom of the swimming pool
- Force pushes humeral head through inferior aspect of joint

Clinical presentation:
- Pain
- Arm held in abduction above head; *luxatio erecta*
- Neurovascular signs; loss of circulation and sensation to upper arm/axilla

Radiographic appearance:
- Head of humerus inferiorly displaced below glenoid fossa
- Humerus abducted more than 90°
- Look for associated fractures to shoulder girdle including greater tuberosity, acromion and coracoid processes, glenoid rim, and clavicle (may be best visualised post-reduction)

Glenohumeral Joint Subluxations

As well as complete dislocations, subluxations may also occur in the same directions as a result of underlying soft tissue injury to the rotator cuff or joint capsule, either acute or chronic, and sometimes associated with other bone injury.

Fig 5.15 Inferior dislocation; luxatio erecta. The humeral head is displaced inferiorly (arrow) to lie inferior to the glenoid (G). The humerus is abducted to more than 90°, which is typical of this form of dislocation. Note that no associated bony injury is demonstrated on this projection. (Source: Diagnostic Imaging: Musculoskeletal, STATdx © Elsevier.)

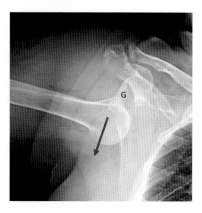

There will only be partial loss of apposition between the articular surface of the humeral head and glenoid fossa. The humeral head may appear displaced inferiorly to its normal articulation with the glenoid fossa, and the sub-acromial distance will be increased.

Greater Tuberosity Avulsion Fracture

(Figs. 5.13, 5.16, and 5.17)

Fractures of the greater tuberosity may occur as isolated fractures or in combination with other injuries such as comminuted fractures of the proximal humerus or glenohumeral joint dislocations.

They may be obvious if there is displacement but also very subtle (or occult) on radiographs, so it is important the greater tuberosity is carefully assessed, particularly on the AP with the arm in external rotation (Fig. 5.2).

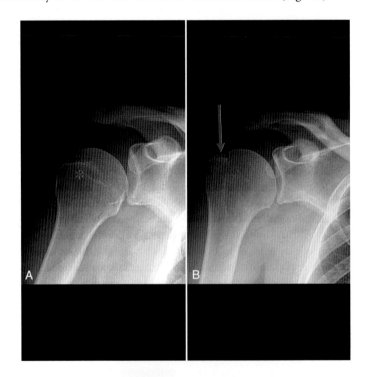

Fig 5.16 Greater tuberosity fracture. Importance of external rotation of the arm. **A,** Internal rotation: note the greater tuberosity is not seen in profile as it lies anteriorly (*) and the fracture not clearly evident. Also note how the rounded appearance of the humeral head mimic a posterior dislocation. **B,** External rotation: the greater tuberosity is in profile and the avulsion fracture demonstrated (arrow). (Source: Diagnostic Imaging: Musculoskeletal, STATdx © Elsevier.)

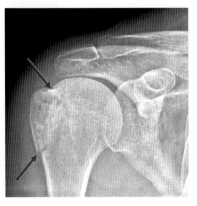

Fig 5.17 Greater tuberosity fracture. This more subtle fracture demonstrates cortical steps of the greater tuberosity superiorly and inferiorly (arrows). (Source: Diagnostic Imaging: Musculoskeletal, STATdx © Elsevier.)

Typical mechanism of injury:
- Isolated avulsion fractures typically following fall; avulsion caused by traction of rotator cuff tendons or due to compression against the acromion
- Variable if other injuries involved (e.g. dislocation)

Clinical presentation:
- Shoulder pain following fall
- Reduced range of movement; unable to abduct arm
- May present clinically very similar to rotator cuff tear

Radiographic appearance:
- Isolated avulsion best demonstrated on AP with arm in internal rotation
- Subtle cortical step/lucent line extending through greater tuberosity
- Overlying soft tissue swelling
- Assess for fracture particularly if presents with anterior/inferior dislocation

Proximal Humeral Fractures

(Figs. 5.18–5.20)

Fractures to the proximal humerus most commonly affect the surgical neck of humerus (the proximal metaphysis) as the weakest part but may also produce comminuted fractures also involving the greater and lesser tuberosities, head, and diaphysis.

Fig 5.18 Proximal humerus fractures. A, one-part fracture; there is an impacted comminuted fracture (several separate small fragments) through the surgical neck of humerus (arrows). It demonstrates no displacement, making this a one-part fracture. **B,** three-part fracture dislocation. There are displaced fractures of the surgical neck (1), shaft (2), and lesser tuberosities (3) of the humerus, making this a three-part fracture. There is also a non-displaced fracture of the greater tuberosity (arrowhead). All of these are in addition to an anterior dislocation. (Source: Diagnostic Imaging: Musculoskeletal, STATdx © Elsevier.)

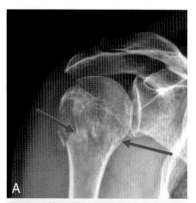
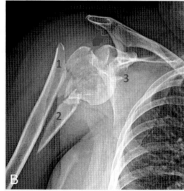

Fig 5.19 Proximal humerus fracture.
Transverse fracture (arrowheads) of the surgical neck of humerus with lateral displacement (arrow). The displacement makes this a two-part fracture. Note the reduced bone density (osteopaenia) on the AP projection. These fractures are most common in the elderly with osteoporosis.

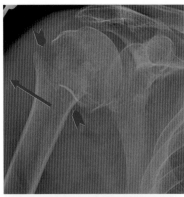

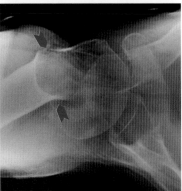

A common (and simple) classification system (the Neer classification) for these types of fractures is based upon the number of fragments produced:

- one-part; undisplaced fracture normally of the surgical neck (most common)
- two-part; single fracture, normally of the surgical neck, with displacement between the head and shaft
- three-part; two fractures, normally the surgical neck and greater tuberosity (sometimes lesser) with displacement
- four-part; three fractures, normally the surgical neck and both tuberosities with displacement

Simple undisplaced fractures are often treated conservatively, whilst more highly comminuted fractures may require surgical intervention or hemiarthroplasty (replacement of the humeral head and neck).

Typical mechanism of injury:

- FOOSH, particularly in elderly; often with arm abducted from side
- High-velocity trauma in younger patients

Clinical presentation:

- Pain and reduced range of movement
- Prominent bruising
- Swelling or deformity of shoulder
- Most common in elderly patients with osteoporosis

Fig 5.20 Proximal humerus fracture. There is an oblique fracture of the neck of the humerus (arrowhead) with lateral and anterior displacement (arrows). Note the normal physeal plates of the humeral head and coracoid process (curved arrows) in this paediatric patient. (Source: Diagnostic Imaging: Musculoskeletal, STATdx © Elsevier.)

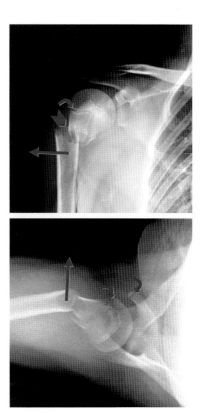

Radiographic appearance:
- Depends on number of fragments
- Surgical neck fracture most common; oblique lucent line traversing proximal humerus. May be impacted.
- Assess for fractures of greater and lesser tuberosities
- Assess for degree of displacement and angulation
- May demonstrate reduced bone density (osteopaenia), since common with underlying osteoporosis
- Soft tissue swelling over lateral head of humerus
- May demonstrate lipohaemarthrosis (horizontal fluid level; see Chapter 6, page 158) in sub-acromial space with inferior subluxation of humeral head

Scapula Fractures
(Figs. 5.21–5.23)

Fractures to the body of the scapula are normally a result of high-velocity injuries and chest trauma. As a result, they are very commonly associated with significant injuries such as pneumothorax, lung contusions, and neurovascular and head injuries.

More often than not they will co-exist with other fractures of the humerus, ribs, or clavicle, which are more likely to fracture than the scapula, so satisfaction of search is essential.

Fig 5.21 Scapula fracture. Comminuted fracture of the body and neck of the scapula (arrows). Note the subtle lucent line which extends into the glenohumeral joint (curved arrows). Axial CT helps to assess the complexity of the injury. (Source: Diagnostic Imaging: Musculoskeletal, STATdx © Elsevier.)

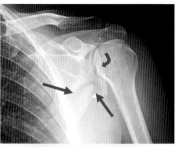

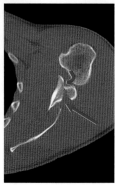

Fig 5.22 Scapula fracture. Fracture involving the body (arrows) and neck (curved arrow) inferior to the glenoid. (Source: Diagnostic Imaging: Musculoskeletal, STATdx © Elsevier.)

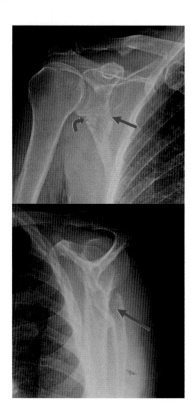

Fig 5.23 Scapula fracture. Vertically orientated fracture through the neck extending from the suprascapular notch (arrow) to the lateral border inferior to the glenoid (curved arrow). Note the associated comminuted clavicle fracture (arrowhead); scapula fractures are commonly seen alongside other injuries. (Source: Diagnostic Imaging: Musculoskeletal, STATdx © Elsevier.)

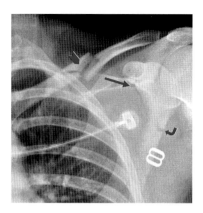

Fractures to the body (most common), neck, and glenoid are often subtle and undisplaced and may well be missed. Overlying anatomy (such as the ribs) can make visualisation difficult, so it is important to assess the scapula carefully. They are often comminuted, and it is important to assess for extension of the fracture into the glenohumeral joint.

Typical mechanism of injury:
- High velocity, for example, road traffic collisions
- Direct blow, for example, hit with a heavy object such as a baseball bat

Clinical presentation:
- Pain over scapula; may be masked by other injuries
- Unable to abduct arm
- Patient often presents with other significant injuries; may be imaged with chest X-ray or CT first

Radiographic appearance:
- AP projection:
  - Usually minimally displaced
  - Look for lucent line in body and cortical step to border
  - Assess lateral border and glenoid in particular; typically involve junction of body and glenoid below glenohumeral joint
  - Often comminuted
  - Assess for extension into glenoid fossa
  - Satisfaction of search; look for other fractures of ribs, clavicle, and humerus and for lung pathology (pneumothorax, opacities)
- Lateral scapula (Y-view) projection:
  - Assess for fractures of body and displacement; cortical step
  - Review other areas, e.g. ribs, chest for pathology

Acromion and Coracoid Process Fractures

Whilst these injuries often occur with other injuries to the shoulder girdle (e.g. dislocations and scapula fractures), they can also occur in isolation either as avulsion fractures or due to direct blows such as in sports.

Often best evaluated on an axial/modified axial projection, fractures appear as separate bone fragments from the rest of the scapula. Care must be taken, particularly in paediatrics and young adults (up to age of around 25 when they fuse; Fig. 5.9), not to confuse the normal ossification centre (or os acromiale) with a fracture.

Acromioclavicular Joint Subluxation/ Dislocation

(Figs. 5.24–5.26)

The AC joint is a natural weak point in the shoulder girdle and therefore is prone to injury, particularly in sports. The joint between the distal clavicle and the acromion process is supported by two sets of ligaments:

- *Coracoclavicular*; two ligaments (conoid and trapezoid) between the coracoid process and inferior part of the clavicle (conoid tubercle). Integral to stability of AC joint injuries
- *Coracoacromial*; between distal clavicle and acromion. Support AC joint but less critical in terms of stability of AC joint injuries

These sets of ligaments (particularly the coracoclavicular) provide stability and an anchor for the rest of the shoulder girdle and upper limb. The stability and severity of AC joint injuries are determined by their involvement.

There are a range of injuries classified (using the Rockwood classification Fig. 5.24) by the involvement of the ligaments and displacement of the clavicle:

Fig 5.24 Rockwood Classification of AC joint injuries. Demonstrate involvement of the acromioclavicular (arrow) and coracoclavicular (arrowhead) ligaments as well as the position of the distal clavicle (curved arrow). (Source: Diagnostic Imaging: Musculoskeletal, STATdx © Elsevier.)

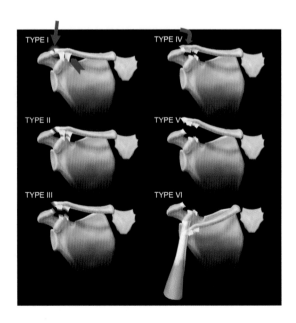

Fig 5.25 AC joint injury.
A, Type II injury; there is loss of the normal acromioclavicular alignment (dotted line) with superior subluxation of the distal clavicle (arrow), but the coracoclavicular distance is within normal limits (arrowhead). **B,** Type III injury; there is loss of the normal acromioclavicular alignment (dotted line) with superior dislocation of the distal clavicle (arrow) and widening of the coracoclavicular distance (arrowhead). (Source: Diagnostic Imaging: Musculoskeletal, STATdx © Elsevier.)

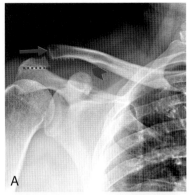

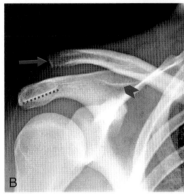

Type	Acromioclavicular Ligaments	Coracoclavicular Ligaments	Distal Clavicle
I	Sprained	Intact	Not displaced
II	Ruptured	Sprained	Not displaced
III	Ruptured	Ruptured	Superior subluxation
IV	Ruptured	Ruptured	Posterior dislocation
V	Ruptured	Ruptured	Superior dislocation
VI	Ruptured	Ruptured	Inferior dislocation

The significance/severity of the injuries increases with the classification. Types IV–VI are more significant, as they also involve detachment of the trapezius and deltoid muscles, but are rarer than types I–III. To assess these injuries on an AP projection we can assess the AC joint space and alignment, as well as the coracoclavicular distance and position of the distal end of clavicle relative to the acromion.

Typical mechanism of injury:
- Fall onto tip of shoulder (acromion); most common. Sports injuries such as in rugby
- FOOSH
- Forced traction of upper limb

Fig 5.26 AC joint injury – Type IV, posterior dislocation. A, The AP projection appears to demonstrate narrowing of the AC joint (arrow) compared to normal but alignment is maintained (dotted line). **B,** The axial projection, however, shows that the distal clavicle (C) is dislocated posteriorly to the acromion process (A). (Source: Diagnostic Imaging: Musculoskeletal, STATdx © Elsevier.)

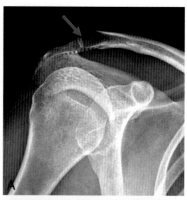

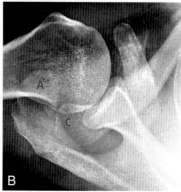

Clinical presentation:
- Pain over AC joint
- 'Clunk' on abducting arm
- Prominence/deformity of distal clavicle
- Most common in young male adults
- Rare in elderly/children due to altered relative bone strength (more prone to fracture)

Radiographic appearance:
- Dependent on severity
- Important to assess for associated fractures
- As per Rockwood classification (Fig. 5.24 and table below):

Type	AC Joint Space	AC Joint Alignment	Coracoclavicular Distance	Position of Distal Clavicle
I	Normal	Normal	Normal	Not displaced
II	Widened	Slightly abnormal	Normal	Not displaced
III	Widened	Abnormal	Widened (<25 mm)	Superiorly subluxed (not above acromion)
IV	May appear normal/narrowed	May appear normal	May appear normal	Posteriorly dislocated

Type	AC Joint Space	AC Joint Alignment	Coracoclavicular Distance	Position of Distal Clavicle
V	Widened	Abnormal	Widened (>25 mm)	Superior dislocation
VI	Widened	Abnormal (in opposite direction)	Narrowed (but in opposite direction)	Inferior dislocation; inferior to coracoid process

Sternoclavicular Joint Dislocation

(Fig. 5.27)

As with fractures of the scapula, dislocations of the SC joint are commonly associated with significant trauma and other underlying soft tissue injury such as pneumothorax, haemothorax, rib fractures, and trauma to the great vessels, mediastinum, and trachea.

Despite being best imaged using CT, it is important to assess the integrity of the SC joint on chest and shoulder radiographs following significant trauma. In young adults, a fracture through the medial clavicle physeal plate may occur instead of dislocation.

Typical mechanism of injury:
- High-velocity direct blow; for example, road traffic collision or sports injury

Clinical presentation:
- Pain; may be masked by other injuries
- Swelling/deformity over SC joint
- Patient often presents with other significant injuries; may be imaged with chest X-ray or CT first

Radiographic appearance:
- May not be visible on radiographs (CT best imaging modality)
- Displacement of medial end of clavicle on sternum (normally superiorly)
- Satisfaction of search; look for other fractures of ribs, clavicle, and humerus and for lung pathology (pneumothorax, opacities)

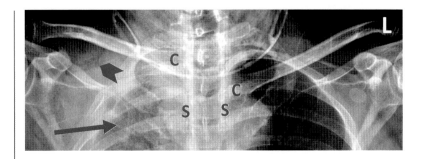

Fig 5.27 Sternoclavicular dislocation. There is superior dislocation of the medial end of the right clavicle (C) on the sternum (S) compared to the left on this supine chest X-ray following a road traffic collision. Also note the opacity in the right hemithorax (arrow) caused by a haemothorax and subcutaneous emphysema (arrowhead) caused by air in the soft tissues. (Source: Diagnostic Imaging: Musculoskeletal, STATdx © Elsevier.)

CLAVICLE

Although visualised on an AP shoulder projection, suspected clavicle injuries should be imaged using dedicated projections, normally the AP and inferosuperior axial. The AP projection should be assessed using a lot of the same criteria as the AP shoulder. The axial projection specifically provides an alternative view of the clavicle bone for fractures.

Systematic Approach

Radiographic appearances of the clavicle (Fig. 5.28)

AP/inferosuperior projections

Follow the standard approach to the AABCSS in addition to:

Adequacy	• Ensure both the AC and SC joints are visualised
Alignment	• AC joint – inferior surfaces of acromion and distal clavicle along same line; any steps/interruptions (AP only)? • Does the medial end of the clavicle articulate with the sternum?
Bones	• Follow the cortex and assess the internal structure of clavicle • Assess other bones visualised on images

Cartilage (Joint spaces)	• AP projection:
	  • AC joint space – is it widened (~8 mm maximum)?
	  • Coracoclavicular distance – is it widened (~12 mm maximum)?

Soft tissues	• Any evidence of soft tissue swelling?
	• Assess the visible chest:
	  • Do the lung markings reach the chest wall?
	  • Is there a visible lung edge – particularly in the apex?
	  • Any evidence of increased opacity in the lung?

Significant areas	• Look for subtle fractures in the mid- and medial clavicle where superimposed by the ribs

Clavicle Fractures

(Fig. 5.29)

Fractures of the clavicle are among the most common, particularly in paediatrics. They make up approximately 5% of all fractures, half of which occur under the age of 10.

Most fracture in the middle third, and the weight of the shoulder girdle causes inferior displacement, so they are readily visible. However, some may be undisplaced and subtle. Fractures to the distal end are less common, and those to the medial end the least common.

Although often without significant complication, displaced fractures, or where there is a high-energy injury, may be associated with other underlying injury such as rib fractures, pneumothorax, or neurovascular injury. Fractures which are displaced may be prone to mal/non-union.

Typical mechanism of injury:
- Fall onto shoulder, for example, sports injury
- FOOSH
- Direct blow

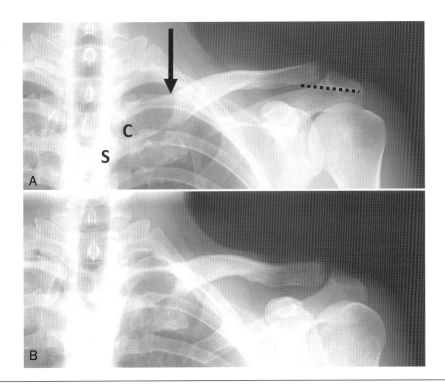

Fig 5.28 Clavicle AP (A) and axial (B) projections: systematic approach. Adequacy – both AC and SC joints included. Alignment – AP only – AC joint alignment (dotted line); medial end of clavicle (C) with sternum (S). Bones – assess clavicle; all other visualised bones; ribs, humerus, scapula. Cartilage – AP only: AC joint space; coracoclavicular distance. Soft tissues – is there any soft tissue swelling? Assess visible chest: do the lung markings reach the chest wall? Is there a visible lung edge – particularly in the apex? Any evidence of increased opacity in the lung? Significant areas – subtle fractures of mid- and medial clavicle (arrow) where superimposed by ribs. (Source: Merrill's Atlas of Radiographic Positioning & Procedures, Fifteenth Edition, 2023.)

Fig 5.29 Clavicle fracture.
There is a comminuted fracture of the mid-clavicle within inferior displacement (arrow). Note the AC joint and coracoclavicular distance are normal, suggesting integrity of the supporting ligaments. (Source: Diagnostic Imaging: Musculoskeletal, STATdx © Elsevier.)

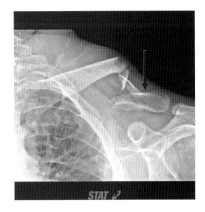

Clinical presentation:
- Pain over clavicle
- Deformity/prominence over fracture
- Most commonly in paediatrics and young adults

Radiographic appearance:
- Usually involved middle third of clavicle; need to assess entire length
- May range from subtle undisplaced fracture to comminuted and displaced fracture
- Displacement usually inferior, or with angulation, and the apex pointed superiorly
- Assess AC joint alignment and coracoclavicular distance for integrity of AC joint and coracoclavicular ligaments
- Satisfaction of search; look for other fractures of ribs, clavicle, and humerus and for lung pathology (pneumothorax, opacities)

LOWER LIMB 6

In this chapter we will consider the interpretation of skeletal radiographs of the lower limb (note that the hip joint and proximal femur are considered separately in Chapter 7). The lower limb is extremely prone to injury due to its extrinsic position and forces placed upon it, particularly in falls and sports injuries.

FEMUR

The femur is the largest bone in the body. As a large long bone, fractures are usually fairly obvious and a typical systematic approach should identify them; however, you should be mindful to review the entire image.

Systematic Approach

Radiographic appearances of the femur (Fig. 6.1)

Anteroposterior and lateral projections

Follow the standard approach to the AABCSS in addition to:

Adequacy	• Are both the hip and knee joint included on the images?
	• Is there overlap between the images if not possible to include on one image?
Alignment	• Are the bones of the hip and knee joints grossly aligned (remember these are not dedicated projections)?
	• Are the hip and knee joint grossly AP/lateral with each other (i.e. no rotation between them)?
Bones	• Assess the femur in its entirety
	• Assess the visible pelvis (e.g. pubic rami) and proximal tibia/fibula and patella
Cartilage (Joint spaces)	• Not dedicated views, difficult to assess joint spaces
	• Is there any gross widening (diastasis)?
Soft tissues	• Is there soft tissue swelling?
	• Evidence of lipohaemarthrosis on lateral (if horizontal beam) – see page 158
Significant areas	• Proximal femur; neck and intertrochanteric regions
	• Do we need dedicated hip/knee projections?

Fig. 6.1 AP and lateral femur projections: systematic approach.
Adequacy – are both hip and knee joints included? Is there overlap between the images? Alignment – are the hip and knee joints grossly AP/lateral with each other (i.e. no rotation between them)? Are the bones of the hip and knee joints grossly aligned? Bones – carefully check ALL of the femur; assess the visible pelvis and tibia/fibula, and patella. Cartilage – difficult to assess joints as not dedicated projections; is there any gross widening? Soft tissues – is there any soft tissue swelling? Evidence of lipohaemarthrosis (if horizontal beam lateral). Significant areas – proximal femur; do we need dedicated hip/knee projections? (Source: Bontrager's Textbook of Radiographic Positioning and Related Anatomy, Tenth Edition, 2021; Radiography Essentials for Limited Practice, Sixth Edition, 2021.)

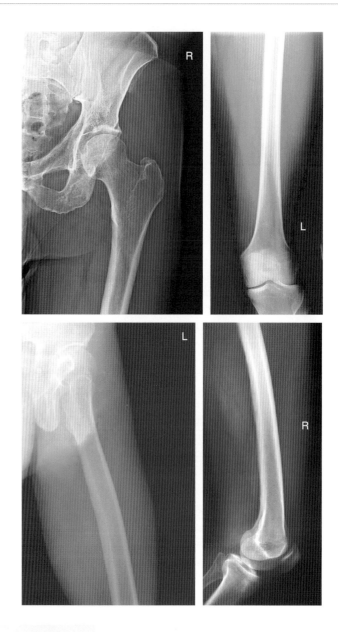

Fractures

As the strongest bone in the body, fractures typically only occur due to high-velocity/high-energy forces or where the bone is weakened due to underlying pathology (e.g. osteoporosis, metastases) or age (paediatrics).

Fractures typically occur either of the shaft (diaphysis) and will be fairly obvious, or proximally around the hip and distally around the knee. The latter 2 are considered when looking at the knee later in this chapter and hip (Chapter 7), respectively, since dedicated projections should be used to assess them.

Shaft/Diaphysis Fracture (Figs. 6.2 and 6.3)

Occur between the subtrochanteric region (5 cm inferior to lesser trochanter) of the proximal femur and supracondylar region of the knee.

Typical mechanism of injury:
- High energy, for example, road traffic collisions
- Pathological due to underlying disease

Clinical presentation:
- Pain, swelling, and foreshortening of leg
- Neurovascular injury possible

Appearance:
- Midshaft; distal to the subtrochanteric region and proximal to the femoral condyles
- Transverse most commonly; may be comminuted oblique or spiral
- Usually obvious due to marked displacement
- Assess for underlying bone pathology

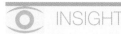 INSIGHT

As with a lot of large long bone fractures, consideration of associated neurovascular injury must be considered due to the close relationship of the femur and femoral artery and sciatic nerve.

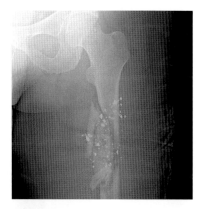

Fig. 6.2 Left femoral fracture. A highly comminuted fracture of the shaft of femur caused by a gunshot with multiple retained metallic foreign bodies. Fractures of the shaft of femur are rarely subtle but are often associated with associated neurovascular injury. (Source: Diagnostic Imaging: Musculoskeletal, STATdx © Elsevier.)

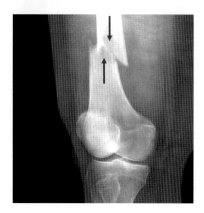

Fig. 6.3 Right femoral pathological fracture. There is an oblique fracture of the distal shaft of femur with lateral displacement. There is a lucency (arrows) within the shaft of the femur on either side of the fracture suggesting this is pathological in nature. This is a bone metastasis. (Source: Diagnostic Imaging: Musculoskeletal, STATdx © Elsevier.)

KNEE

The knee is the largest joint in the body. The demands put upon it, and its extrinsic position, make it prone to injury. Many injuries, particularly in adults, are soft tissue in nature, though a thorough interpretation of radiographs can demonstrate fractures and signs of soft tissue injury.

Following trauma, the anteroposterior and horizontal beam lateral are the standard projections.

Anteroposterior Projection

Adequacy (Fig. 6.4)

Ensure the knee is truly anteroposterior (AP); do not purely rely on the position of the patella to assess rotation, as this can be dislocated/subluxed. Also use the position of the fibula in relation to the tibia and the appearance of the intercondylar eminences (central in intercondylar fossa) to assess for rotation. The knee joint should be extended and the image centred over the joint space (as with all joint radiographs).

Alignment (Fig. 6.4)

Alignment can be assessed in several ways:
- *Patella:* assess whether the position of the patella is central between the medial and lateral femoral condyles
- *Femorotibial alignment 1:* the respective lateral and medial aspects aspect of the femoral and tibial condyles should be aligned
- *Femorotibial alignment 2:* a straight line drawn down the shaft of femur should align with the shaft of the tibia with minimal angulation (narrowing of the medial or lateral joint space due to osteoarthritis may affect this)
- *Fibula head:* approximately one-half should be superimposed by the tibia

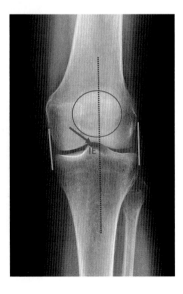

Fig. 6.4 AP knee projections: adequacy and alignment. Adequacy – true AP position: patella central (circle); intercondylar eminences (IE) central within intercondylar fossa (arrow); fibula head (FH) half superimposed by tibia. Centred over joint space; Alignment – patella central (circle); femorotibial alignment: lateral and medial joint surfaces aligned (lines), straight line along shafts of femur/tibia (dotted line). (Source: Bontrager's Textbook of Radiographic Positioning and Related Anatomy, Tenth Edition, 2021.)

Bones (Fig. 6.5)

The bones' external cortex and internal texture should be carefully assessed by looking at the femur, tibia, and fibula including at the edge of the image. Some particular areas to consider:

Patella: assess carefully for lucent line, as subtle fractures may be identified (though not always)

Femoral condyles: review the articular surfaces of each condyle for steps/depressions

Tibial condyles:

- The two tibial plateaus slope slighty inferiorly from anterior to posterior; as such, normally both the anterior and posterior edges can usually be identified separately
- The tibial plateaus should be concave in shape; the slightly more sclerotic central portion can normally be seen
- Loss of either of these two appearances can indicate fracture
- A remnant of the proximal tibial epiphyseal plate is often visualised as a thin horizontal sclerotic line distal to the joint; do not confuse for fracture

Intercondylar eminences: assess both for avulsion fracture (more common in immature skeletons)

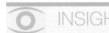 INSIGHT

Remember, the *tibial condyles* (medial and lateral) are the two widened masses of bone at the proximal end of the tibia. The *tibial plateaus* are the flattened articular surfaces on the tibial condyles.

Fig. 6.5 AP knee projections: bones.
Femur, tibia, fibula (including edges of image); patella (P); articular surfaces of femoral condyles (arrows); tibial condyles: separate anterior/posterior edges (solid lines), concavity centrally (dotted line); intercondylar eminences for avulsion (hollow arrow); note the normal remnant of tibial physeal plate (curved arrow). (Source: Bontrager's Textbook of Radiographic Positioning and Related Anatomy, Tenth Edition, 2021.)

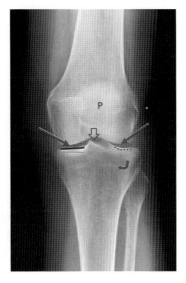

Cartilage (Fig. 6.6)

It is important to look carefully within the joint spaces to identify any small avulsion fractures/osteochondral fracture fragments which lie within the joint.

No clear joint space between the proximal tibia and fibula should be seen.

Soft Tissues (Fig. 6.6)

Assess for generalised soft tissue swelling as well as focal swelling adjacent to the medial and lateral joint lines.

Significant Areas
(Fig. 6.6)

There are some subtle fractures that occur related to the knee joint that should be carefully looked for. Hopefully the assessment already described will identify this but specifically assess:

- The patella for subtle lucent fracture lines
- The intercondylar eminences for avulsion (particularly in paediatric patients)
- The articular surfaces of the femoral condyles
- The tibial plateaus
- The tip of the head of fibula, lateral to the tibial condyle for small bone fragments
- The bones at the edge of the image

Fig. 6.6 AP knee projections: cartilage, soft tissues, and significant areas.
Cartilage: assess joint space for intraarticular fragments; joint space widening/narrowing. Soft tissues: general soft tissue swelling, medial/lateral joint swelling (hollow arrows). Significant areas: patella, intercondylar eminences, femoral condyle articular surfaces, tibial plateaus, tip of fibula head/lateral aspect lateral tibial condyle (arrow). (Source: Bontrager's Textbook of Radiographic Positioning and Related Anatomy, Tenth Edition, 2021.)

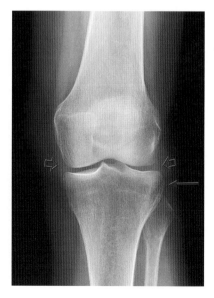

Systematic Approach   Radiographic appearances of the knee joint, AP projection (Figs. 6.4–6.6)

Anteroposterior projection

Follow the standard approach to the AABCSS in addition to:

Adequacy	• True AP position:
	    • Patella central
	    • Intercondylar eminences central
	    • One-half fibula head superimposed by tibia
	• Image centred over joint

Alignment	• Patella; central
	• Femorotibial alignment:
	    • Lateral and medial joint surfaces aligned
	    • Straight line along shafts of femur and tibia
	• Fibula head superimposed by tibia

Bones	• Assess the femur, tibia, and fibula in turn (including edge of image)
	• Patella for fracture lines
	• Articular surface of medial/lateral femoral condyles
	• Tibial condyles:
	    • Anterior/posterior edges of medial/lateral tibial plateau
	    • Medial/lateral tibial plateaus concave centrally
	• Intercondylar eminences, ?avulsion fracture

Cartilage (Joint spaces)	• Assess for presence of intra-articular bone fragments
Soft tissues	• Soft tissue swelling, especially over medial lateral joint
Significant areas	• Patella • Intercondylar eminences • Femoral condyle articular surfaces • Tibial plateaus • Tip of fibula head/lateral aspect lateral tibial condyle

Lateral (Horizontal Beam) Projection

The lateral projection following trauma is normally undertaken with the patient supine, the leg in a horizontal position and with a horizontal X-ray beam rather than with the patient laying their side. This is predominantly to allow visualisation of soft tissue signs, the *lipohaemarthrosis*, which will only be visualised in this position, though it may also be considered more comfortable for the patient following injury.

Adequacy (Fig. 6.7)   Ensure the image has been undertaken in horizontal position; it should be annotated on the image. This normally results in the knee being extended or in minimal flexion.

The femoral condyles should be superimposed to allow clear visualisation of the patellofemoral and femorotibial joint spaces and the intercondylar eminences and posterior cortex of the patella (sites of subtle fracture).

The area of interest must include sufficient of the distal femur to ensure the suprapatellar bursa is included.

Fig. 6.7 Lateral Knee Projection: Adequacy and Alignment. Adequacy – Is it a horizontal beam lateral (annotation)? Are the femoral condyles superimposed (dotted lines)? Are the patellofemoral and femorotibial joint spaces clear (arrows)? Alignment – Are the femoral condyles (dotted lines) articulating with the tibial plateaus (solid lines)? Does the posterior surface of the patella (P) articulate with the rounded articular surface of the femoral condyles (dotted lines)? (Source: DeLee, Drez, & Miller's Orthopaedic Sports Medicine: Principles and Practice , Fifth Edition, 2020).

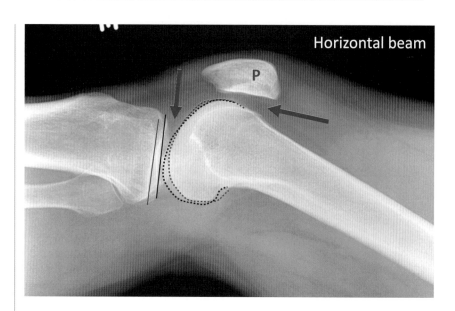

Horizontal beam

Alignment (Fig. 6.7)

The posterior surface of the patella should articulate with the anterior rounded aspect of the femoral condyles; significant displacement may indicate rupture of the quadriceps tendon (the patella will displace inferiorly) or the patella tendon (patella displaces superiorly).

Bones (Fig. 6.8)

The bones' external cortex and internal texture should be carefully assessed by looking at the patella, femur, tibia, and fibula including at the edge of the image. Some particular areas to consider:

Patella: assess carefully for lucent line as subtle fractures may be identified, particularly on the anterior and posterior cortex

Femoral condyles: review the rounded articular surfaces of each condyle for steps/depressions (note there is a normal shallow depression on the flattened distal aspect of the lateral femoral condyle)

Tibial plateaus:

- The two tibial plateaus slope slightly inferiorly (by approximately up to 10°) from anterior to posterior
- Follow the cortex of each of the two tibial plateaus
- Loss of either of these two appearances can indicate fracture.
- A remnant of the tibial tuberosity is often visualised anteriorly on the tibia (especially in adolescents and young adults) and should not be confused with fracture (which is rare).
- Also assess bone just distal to the tibial plateaus for fracture line (lucent/sclerotic line), but again remember the normal remnant of the epiphyseal plate

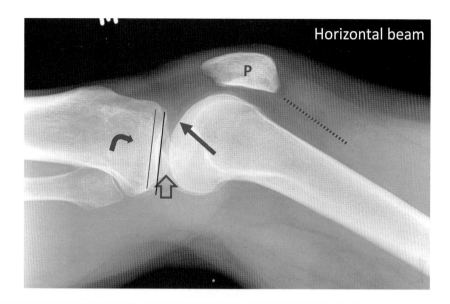

Fig. 6.8 Lateral Knee Projection: Bones, cartilage (joints) and soft tissues. Bones – Assess the femur, tibia, and fibula (including edge of image); Patella (P) for fracture lines; especially anterior and posterior surface; Articular surface of femoral condyles – notice the normal slight flattening/concavity of the lateral condyle (arrow); Tibial plateaus (solid lines); Two separate continuous lines; Slope inferiorly from anterior to posterior; Intercondylar eminences/spines for avulsion (hollow arrow); Note the normal remnant of the epiphyseal growth plate (curved arrow). Cartilage – Assess for intraarticular bone fragments. Soft tissues – General soft tissue swelling, especially anteriorly; Assess suprapatellar bursa which is normally not visible (dotted line indicates position). (Source: DeLee, Drez, & Miller's Orthopaedic Sports Medicine: Principles and Practice, Fifth Edition, 2020.)

Intercondylar eminences: assess for avulsion fractures (more common in immature skeletons)

Be mindful of the other common sesamoid bone in the knee (besides the patella) called the *fabella*, which lies in the lateral head of gastrocnemius tendon. Where present, this smooth round osseous density lies posterior to the femoral condyles and should not be confused for fracture.

Cartilage (Fig. 6.8)

It is important to look carefully within the joint spaces to identify any small avulsion fractures/osteochondral fracture fragments which lie within the joint.

Soft Tissues

(Figs. 6.8–6.10)

Soft tissue swelling, particularly over the anterior surface of the knee, can be an indicator of injury. Perhaps of more significance is the presence of fluid within the suprapatellar bursa, either *effusion* or *lipohaemarthrosis*, in a complex but important principle that requires some explanation.

Fig. 6.9 Suprapatellar effusion. There is fusiform (sausage-shaped) soft tissue opacity in the region of the suprapatellar bursa in keeping with an effusion. (Source: Diagnostic Imaging: Musculoskeletal, STATdx © Elsevier.)

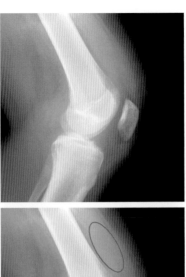
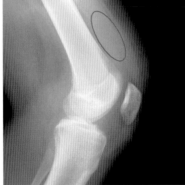

Effusion (Fig. 6.9)

The suprapatellar bursa is a recess of the synovial membrane connected directly to the main part of the knee joint. Normally it contains a trace amount of synovial fluid to help allow friction-free movement of the quadriceps tendon against the femur, but the amount of fluid can increase (an effusion) following trauma and/or pathology (see Chapter 2, page 28). This distends the bursa, which can then often be seen radiographically on a lateral projection as a 'sausage-shaped' opacity superior to the patella.

Following trauma, this fluid is most likely to be blood (and called a *haemarthrosis*), either from soft tissue or bony injury, but the presence of effusion is not indicative of a definite fracture.

Lipohaemarthrosis (Fig. 6.10)

In a fracture of the knee where the fracture extends into the joint (i.e. the tibial plateau, posterior surface of patella, and femoral condyles), this fracture allows both blood and fatty bone marrow to enter the joint capsule.

Like oil and water, blood and fatty bone marrow do not mix. If we immobilise the leg in a horizontal position, then it allows the blood and fatty bone marrow to separate and rise to the highest point in the joint, that is, the suprapatellar bursa.

Fig. 6.10 Lipohaemar-
throsis. There is a fusiform
opacity in the suprapatellar
bursa (circle) with a central
horizontal fluid level (solid
line) where the more lucent
fat lies on top of the more
opaque blood. A very subtle
femoral condyle fracture
(arrow) is evident which was
not visible on the AP projection and may well have
been missed without the
lipohaemarthrosis indicating
a definite intraarticular fracture was present. (Source:
Diagnostic Imaging:
Musculoskeletal, STATdx
© Elsevier.)

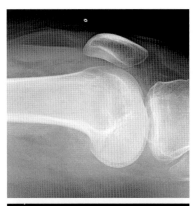

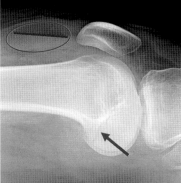

A horizontal beam lateral projection will demonstrate this separation as a
fluid level/line. Where present, this indicates there must be an intra-articular
fracture present and is an extremely useful sign where subtle/occult fracture
lines are present.

Whilst useful, this sign does come with some pitfalls/considerations:

- It will only be evident on a horizontal beam lateral (and given time for
  the fluid to separate); a turned lateral will not demonstrate the fluid
  level, though it may still show an effusion.
- A positive lipohaemarthrosis indicates a definite intra-articular fracture,
  but a lack of the sign does not rule out a fracture:
  - Rupture to the joint capsule will mean the fluid will dissipate else-
    where in the soft tissues.
  - The fracture might not be intra-articular (e.g. of the tibial/femoral
    shaft), and therefore the fluid will not collect in the joint capsule.

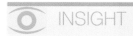 INSIGHT

In Summary

Effusion: demonstrated as fluid opacity in the suprapatellar bursa on both turned and horizontal beam laterals. Following trauma, this *suggests* an intra-articular injury (either bone or soft tissue) and should raise suspicion, but it may be due to another cause (e.g. arthritis or infection). May also occur in other joints in the body (e.g. elbow, ankle)

  Lipohaemarthrosis: demonstrated as a horizontal fluid level/line in the suprapatellar bursa on a horizontal beam lateral but not a turned lateral (may appear as an effusion, though). Indicates a *definite intra-articular* fracture is present and warrants further investigation. Most common in the knee but also sometimes seen in the shoulder.

  The absence of effusion/lipohaemarthrosis does *not* rule out injury.

Significant Areas

Sites of commonly missed or subtle injuries which warrant additional consideration and a second look are:

- The posterior articular surface of the patella
- The tibial plateaus
- The intercondylar eminences
- The neck of fibula on the edge of the image

Systematic Approach

Radiographic appearances of the knee joint, lateral projection (Figs. 6.7 and 6.8)

Lateral projection

Follow the standard approach to the AABCSS in addition to:

Adequacy	• Is it a horizontal beam lateral? • Are the joint spaces clear?
Alignment	• Does the articular surface of the patella articulate with the round femoral condyles? Is it displaced superiorly/inferiorly? • Is the tibia articulating with the femur?

Bones	• Assess the femur, tibia, and fibula in turn (including edge of image)
	• Patella for fracture lines; especially anterior/posterior surface
	• Articular surface of femoral condyles
	• Tibial plateaus:
	  • Two separate continuous lines
	  • Slope inferiorly by up to 10°
	• Intercondylar eminences, ?avulsion fracture

Cartilage (Joint spaces)	• Assess for presence of intra-articular bone fragments in both the patellofemoral and femorotibial joints

Soft tissues	• Soft tissue swelling, especially anteriorly
	• Assess the suprapatellar bursa:
	  • Is there an opacity (effusion)?
	  • Is there a horizontal fluid line (lipohaemarthrosis)?

Significant areas	• Posterior surface of the patella • The tibial plateaus • Intercondylar eminences • Neck of fibula

Fractures/Trauma

As indicated, the knee is extremely prone to injury, both bony and soft tissue. Complex fractures can be fully assessed on CT, and soft tissue injuries are best visualised on MRI, but on knee radiographs a number of fractures may be seen, including:

- Fractures of the distal femur/condyles
- Fractures of the tibial plateau/condyles
- Fractures of the patella
- Osteochondral fractures
- Avulsion fractures, in particular:
  - Segond fractures
  - The intercondylar eminences
- Dislocations:
  - Knee joint
  - Patella

Distal Femur Fractures

(Figs. 6.10–6.12)

Fractures of the condyles of the distal femur may occur in a range of different fracture patterns depending on their location and fracture orientation such as:

- Supracondylar; horizontal fracture superior to the condyles
- T or Y shaped; horizontal fracture (as per the supracondylar above) with a sagittal (vertical) fracture between the two condyles
- Unicondylar only involving the medial or lateral condyle

Fig. 6.11 Femoral condyle fractures. These images display the typical orientation of distal femur fractures that may occur. They may involve one condyle, both condyles, or the supracondylar region (arrows). (Source: Diagnostic Imaging: Musculoskeletal, STATdx © Elsevier.)

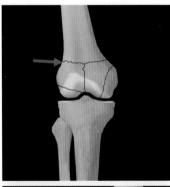

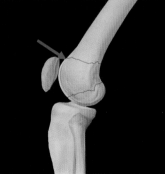

Fig. 6.12 Comminuted distal femur fracture.
There is a fracture of the supracondylar region (arrows) of the femur with posterior displacement of the knee on the lateral. (Source: Diagnostic Imaging: Musculoskeletal, STATdx © Elsevier.)

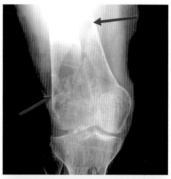

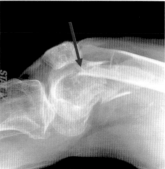

They are relatively uncommon but follow a similar pattern of shaft fractures, occurring due to high-velocity/high-energy forces or where the bone is weakened due to underlying pathology.

Normally they are fairly obvious due to displacement, though not all fracture lines will be evident, depending on the orientation in relation to the X-ray beam, so CT is useful. They may be associated with neurovascular injury.

Typical mechanism of injury:
- High energy, for example, road traffic collisions
- Pathological due to underlying pathology (e.g. osteoporosis)

Clinical presentation:
- Knee pain and swelling
- Neurovascular injury possible

Appearance:
- Usually displaced, though may be subtle dependent on orientation and displacement
- Look for lucent fracture lines on both AP and lateral projections
- Often more than one fracture
- Assess femoral condyles for steps/interruptions
- Often cause lipohaemarthrosis

Tibial Plateau Fractures

(Figs. 6.13–6.15)

Also known as 'bumper' fractures, as they are often seen as a result of pedestrians being struck by a car (the knee is about the height of the bumper). As a result, fractures of the lateral tibial plateau are more common (up to 80%)

because this lateral force drives the femur into the lateral tibial plateau. The lateral tibial plateau is also the weaker of the two.

Whilst they can be extremely obvious due to displacement, they can also be extremely subtle, or even occult, on radiographs, so thorough assessment of the tibial condyles is essential; oblique radiographs of the knee can also be helpful. A lipohaemarthrosis is common in these injuries.

Since these injuries often lead to high levels of morbidity (instability and osteoarthritis), prompt diagnosis and management are essential, and CT is often used for assessment prior to surgery.

The Schatzker classification (Fig. 6.13) is commonly used to grade tibial plateau fractures based upon the type (vertical, depressed, or comminuted) and location (medial, lateral, bicondylar). Unlike a lot of classifications, the higher number does not necessarily indicate severity or prognosis.

Type 3 are the most common but also often the hardest to see!

Schatzger Type	Description	Aetiology
I	Vertical fracture of lateral tibial condyle	Low energy; young adults
II	Vertical fracture and depression of articular surface of lateral condyle	Low energy; elderly/osteoporotic adults
III	Depression fracture of lateral tibial plateau	Low energy; elderly/osteoporotic adults.
IV	Vertical +/− depression fracture of medial tibial plateau; may extend into intercondylar spines	High energy; young adults
V	Bicondylar fracture of medial and lateral tibial condyles	High energy; young adults
VI	Bicondylar fracture with transverse/oblique fracture of metaphysis	High energy; young adults

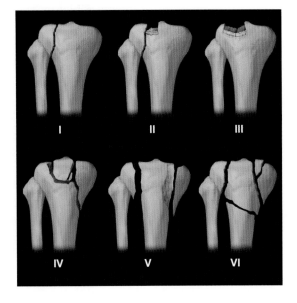

Fig. 6.13 Tibial plateau fractures; the Schatzker classification. (Source: Diagnostic Imaging: Musculoskeletal, STATdx © Elsevier.)

Fig. 6.14 Tibial plateau fracture; Schatzker type II. A, The AP radiograph demonstrates a vertical fracture, or split, of the lateral tibial plateau (arrow) with a possible depressed fragment (hollow arrow). **B,** A coronal CT confirms depression (hollow arrow), making this a split-depression fracture of the lateral tibial condyle – Type II. (Source: Diagnostic Imaging: Musculoskeletal, STATdx © Elsevier.)

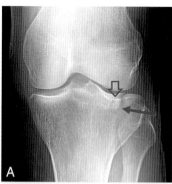

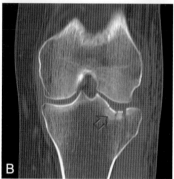

Fig. 6.15 Tibial plateau fracture; Schatzker type III. A, The AP radiograph only demonstrates one side of the lateral tibial plateau (hollow arrow); the other is missing with a very faint sclerotic area within the condyle (arrow). This is typical of type III fracture, which is often very subtle. The lateral projection was normal, with no lipohaemarthrosis. **B,** A sagittal CT confirms depression (arrow) of the lateral tibial plateau. Note the blood (haemarthrosis) in the suprapatellar bursa (curved arrow). (Source: Diagnostic Imaging: Musculoskeletal, STATdx © Elsevier.)

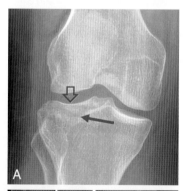

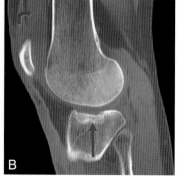

Typical mechanism of injury:
- High energy, for example, road traffic collisions; pedestrian versus car. Lateral force more common than medial
- Low energy; due to fall (in elderly or with underlying osteoporosis)

Clinical presentation:
- Young adults or elderly/with underlying osteoporosis
- Knee pain and swelling
- Unable to weight-bear

Appearance:
- Dependent on type
- Maybe subtle/occult or severely displaced
- Assess for:
  - Longitudinal fracture line (called a split) extending from joint surface and exiting inferior to the condyle
  - Depression fracture; loss of tibial plateau lines/slope and sclerotic area distal to joint surface
- Lateral tibial plateau more common
- Lipohaemarthrosis

Patella Fractures

(Figs. 6.16 and 6.17)

Dependent on the orientation of the fracture, patella fractures can either be markedly displaced or very subtle. Transverse fractures are often displaced due to the traction of the quadriceps and patella tendons if the medial and lateral

Fig. 6.16 Transverse fracture of the patella.
Note the distracted two parts of the patella (arrows) on both projections caused by the pull of the now retracted quadriceps (hollow arrow) and patella (curved arrow) tendons. The displacement indicates rupture of the patella retinaculum which holds the patella in position; otherwise, the fracture would not displace and would be more subtle. (Source: Diagnostic Imaging: Musculoskeletal, STATdx © Elsevier.)

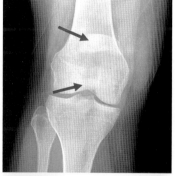
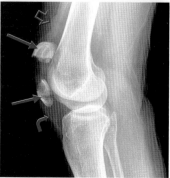

Fig. 6.17 Comminuted (stellate) fracture of the patella. Multiple fracture lines (arrows) are demonstrated on the AP projection **(A)**. The coronal CT **(B)** demonstrates the fractures extend from a central point (hollow arrow) giving rise to the *stellate* (starlike) appearance. The intact supporting soft tissues prevent displacement of the fracture. (Source: Diagnostic Imaging: Musculoskeletal, STATdx © Elsevier.)

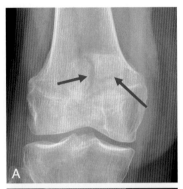

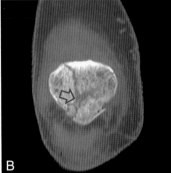

retinaculum (fibrous tissue holding the patella in position) is also ruptured. Vertical/longitudinal fractures often do not displace and may not be visible on either projection.

Typical mechanism of injury:
- Direct blow, for example, fall directly onto knee
- Kicking injury; forced flexion of the knee

Clinical presentation:
- Knee pain and swelling
- Unable to extend knee/reduced strength

Appearance:
- Maybe subtle/occult or severely displaced
- Dependent on type
  - *Longitudinal:* subtle lucent fracture line on AP projection only, often minimally displaced
  - *Transverse:* fracture line on AP and lateral projections, may be minimally or significantly displaced
  - *Comminuted/stellate:* 'star-shaped' fracture lines on AP projection radiating from central point
  - *Avulsion:* small fracture fragment typically of the superior edge
- Lipohaemarthrosis/effusion common

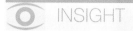

INSIGHT

The *bipartite* (two-part) and, less commonly, *tripartite* (three-part) patella are normal variants representing unfused ossification centres which may be confused with fracture. The secondary ossification centre in the bipartite patella is found on the superolateral surface, has rounded smooth edges, and is smaller than the hole in which it appears to come from and so different in appearance to a fracture (Fig. 6.18).

Osteochondral Fractures

(Figs. 6.19 and 6.20)

Similar to those described in the elbow, fractures of the articular surface of the femoral condyles (though can also affect tibia and patella) comprise both bone and cartilage. They can be both acute, following trauma, and chronic. The chronic form, known as *osteochondritis dissecans* (OCD), is most common in adolescents and affects the medial condyle much more commonly the lateral.

Both are important to diagnose, as they may lead to knee instability and osteoarthritis.

Typical mechanism of injury:

- Acute: either direct injury (e.g. in sports) or indirect such as following patella dislocation (patella fractures the femoral condyle)
- Chronic (OCD): repetitive stress/injury (e.g. due to sports)

Fig. 6.18 Bipartite patella. This normal variant (arrow) is found in the superolateral aspect of the patella, is smooth and round, and smaller than the 'hole' in the patella where it would fit (hollow arrow), and should not be confused with fracture. (Source: Diagnostic Imaging: Musculoskeletal, STATdx © Elsevier.)

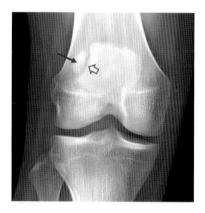

Fig. 6.19 Osteochondral fracture of the medial femoral condyle. There is a very subtle linear bone fragment and defect of the femoral condyle (arrow). Note the small lipohaemarthrosis fluid level (hollow arrow). (Source: Diagnostic Imaging: Musculoskeletal, STATdx © Elsevier.)

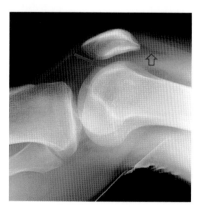

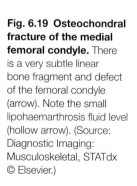

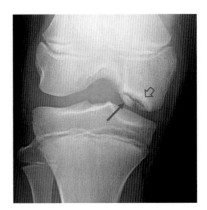

Fig. 6.20 Osteochondritis dissecans (OCD). A smooth bone fragment (arrow) adjacent to a defect in the medial femoral condyle is typical for osteochondritis dissecans. Note the sclerosis (hollow arrow) of the subchondral bone of the defect, which indicates this is chronic. (Source: Diagnostic Imaging: Musculoskeletal, STATdx © Elsevier.)

Clinical presentation:
- Both most common in active/sporty adolescents and young adults
- Pain and swelling
- Knee locking and instability

Appearance:
- Lucency of articular surface of femoral condyle
- Adjacent fragment of bone (though may displace within knee joint)
- Acute:
  - Lipohaemarthrosis/haemarthrosis
  - Typically occur more anteriorly and laterally on femoral condyles (due to impact of patella)
- Chronic (OCD):
  - Usually medial femoral condyle on flattened distal surface
  - Bone appears more rounded, smooth, and sclerotic than in acute fracture
  - May cause effusion (not lipohaemarthrosis)

Avulsion Fractures

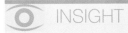 INSIGHT

Avulsion fractures around the knee are commonly associated with other, more significant injuries such as to ligaments and meniscus, and so typically warrant further imaging and investigation.

Due to the number of attachments within and surrounding the knee joint, avulsion fractures are demonstrated at a number of sites. Although they can occur at any age, they are most common in the immature skeleton, as the bones are generally weaker. An avulsion fracture might be considered akin to a ligament rupture, since both result in reduced stability.

Not all avulsion fractures can be visualised on the standard AP/lateral projections; MRI is preferable, as it is also able to assess soft tissue structures. Some of the more commonly avulsion fractures seen on radiographs include:

Anterior (medial) tibial spine/eminence – anterior cruciate ligament (ACL)
Posterior (lateral) tibial spine/eminence – posterior cruciate ligament (PCL)
Adductor tubercle of femur – medial collateral ligament (MCL)
Tip of head of fibula – lateral collateral ligament (LCL) and arcuate ligament
Lateral aspect of lateral tibial condyle (the *Segond* fracture) – anterior longitudinal ligament (ALL)
Apex of patella and tibial tuberosity – patella tendon (proximal and distal insertions)

Tibial Spine/ Eminence Avulsion Fractures (Figs. 6.21 and 6.22)

More common in immature skeletons, such injuries are akin to rupture of the anterior and posterior cruciate ligaments which are more common in the mature skeleton. The medial/anterior tibial spine, which is the insertion of the anterior cruciate ligament (ACL), is more commonly avulsed (as is the ACL more commonly injured). Consideration of associated injury to the meniscus in particular must be made.

Fig. 6.21 Tibial spine avulsion fracture. There is a small avulsion fracture (arrows) of the anterior and medial tibial spine at the insertion of the anterior cruciate ligament in this paediatric. These injuries can be extremely subtle. MRI is probably warranted to look for further injury, such as of the meniscus. (Source: Diagnostic Imaging: Musculoskeletal, STATdx © Elsevier.)

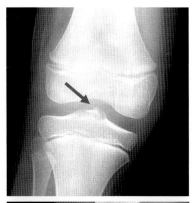
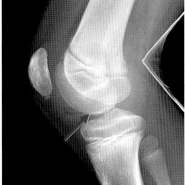

Fig. 6.22 Tibial spine avulsion and Segond fractures. A very small and subtle longitudinal avulsion fracture (arrow) from the lateral tibial condyle, just distal to the joint, is typical of a Segond fracture. Such injuries almost always are associated with other underlying soft tissue injuries, and thus warrant further investigation. A lucency (hollow arrow) in the medial tibial spine indicates an avulsion of the attachment of the anterior cruciate ligament. (Source: Diagnostic Imaging: Musculoskeletal, STATdx © Elsevier.)

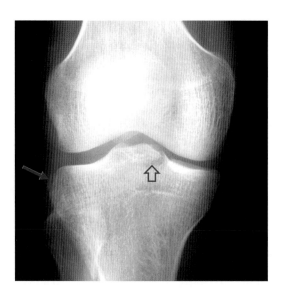

Typical mechanism of injury:
- Twisting injuries; particularly in sports

Clinical presentation:
- Usually older children and adolescents (pre-skeletal maturity)
- Pain and swelling
- Knee instability and locking

Appearance:
- Small linear bone fragment adjacent to site of tibial spines within knee joint
- More common of medial/anterior tibial spine
- Possible lucency/cortical defect in adjacent tibia at site of avulsion
- Lipohaemarthrosis/haemarthrosis

Segond Fracture

(Fig. 6.22)

Described by Paul Segond in 1879, this is an extremely subtle but significant injury. The avulsion fracture caused by the insertion of the anterior longitudinal ligament (ALL) on the lateral aspect of the lateral tibial condyle, just distal to the knee joint, is not particularly significant in itself, but it is associated with other more important injuries such as ACL rupture (in up to 100% of cases) and injury to the meniscus. As such, it is very important to identify on radiographs.

A 'reverse-Segond' fracture on the medial side of the knee at the insertion of the MCL may also be seen but does not normally have the same significance.

Typical mechanism of injury:
- Medial force on flexed knee with foot planted on floor
- Sports injuries, for example, football and skiing

Clinical presentation:
- Pain and swelling
- Knee locking and instability

- Positive anterior drawer, Lachman, and pivot-shift tests (clinical assessment of ACL injuries)

Appearance:

- Classic appearance:
  - Small (<1 cm) longitudinal fracture fragment
  - Adjacent to lateral aspect of lateral tibial condyle, distal to knee joint
- Do not confuse with avulsions of tip of fibula head, which are more distal and usually horizontal
- Haemarthrosis due to soft tissue injury (no lipohaemarthrosis as fracture is outside of the articular capsule)

 INSIGHT

A chronic condition caused by chronic or previous injury to the medial collateral ligament (MCL) should not be mistaken for fracture. *Pellegrini-Stieda disease* (Fig. 6.23), as it is known, causes calcification of the ligament adjacent to the adductor tubercle of the medial femoral condyle and appears more dense than an avulsion fracture (which can also occur at the same place caused by the MCL).

Knee Dislocation

(Fig. 6.24)

Dislocations of the knee joint are extremely significant injuries, as there is a high association with neurovascular injury as well as injury to the cruciate and collateral ligaments and meniscus.

They may also be associated with avulsion fractures or other bony injury, so this should be considered on both pre- (if performed) and post-reduction imaging. They are often reduced prior to imaging due to the risk of neurovascular injury.

Typical mechanism of injury:

- Usually high energy, for example, road traffic collision, fall from height, or sports injury

Clinical presentation:

- Pain, swelling, and deformity
- Instability and loss of function

Fig. 6.23 Pellegrini-Stieda disease. A dense area of longitudinal calcification adjacent to the adductor tubercle can be confused with an avulsion fracture but indicates chronic or previous MCL injury. (Source: Diagnostic Imaging: Musculoskeletal, STATdx © Elsevier.)

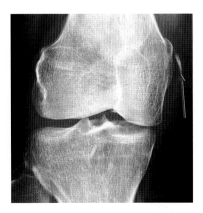

Fig. 6.24 Knee dislocation. There is anterior dislocation of the tibia on the femur. Whilst no associated fractures are visible, there will certainly be significant underlying soft tissue injury. (Source: Diagnostic Imaging: Musculoskeletal, STATdx © Elsevier.)

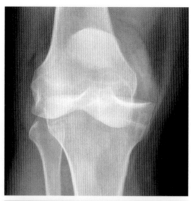
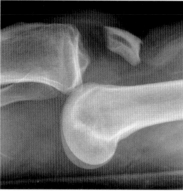

- Loss of foot pulse if popliteal artery injured
- Altered sensation in lower leg due to peroneal nerve injury

Appearance:

- Usually obvious due to gross displacement of tibia on femur
- May occur in any direction
- Superimposition of tibia/femur on one projection, loss of alignment on other
- Assess for associated fractures such as:
  - Avulsions
  - Femoral condyle
  - Tibial plateau
- Will not normally demonstrate haemarthrosis/lipohaemarthrosis as joint capsule most likely to be ruptured and any fluid dissipates

Patella Dislocations

(Fig. 6.25)

Whilst held strongly in place superiorly and inferiorly by the quadriceps and patella tendons, medially and laterally the patella is only fairly weakly supported by the fibrous retinaculum. As such dislocations may occur, normally laterally.

They usually reduce spontaneously when the knee is extended and therefore may not be seen radiographically, though associated avulsion or osteochondral fractures of the femoral condyles may occur where the patella impacts upon them. Patella dislocations are often recurrent and may occur with minimal force.

Fig. 6.25 Patella dislocation (post reduction) and lateral femoral condyle fracture. This patient with a spontaneously reduced dislocation shows normal appearances of the patella. A bone fragment (arrow) within the anterior knee joint and associated subtle lucency/defect (hollow arrows) of the lateral condyle are consistent with an osteochondral fracture caused as the patella dislocated and reduced. Note the lipohaemarthrosis (curved arrow) on the horizontal beam lateral, and the normal appearance of an immature tibial tuberosity (*). (Source: Diagnostic Imaging: Pediatrics, STATdx © Elsevier.)

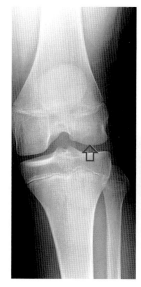
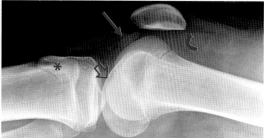

Typical mechanism of injury:
- Twisting injury/direct blow, for example, sports injury
- May be recurrent with minimal force

Clinical presentation:
- Pain and swelling
- History of patella dislocation

Appearance:
- Patella displaced from centre of femur on AP projection (usually lateral), though often normal, as most spontaneously relocate
- Assess for fracture fragments within joint
- Associated lucencies/cortical defect of femoral condyles, particularly over lateral aspect of lateral condyle
- Haemarthrosis or lipohaemarthrosis (if associated fracture)

TIBIA AND FIBULA

As with other long bones such as the humerus and forearm, radiographic evaluation of the lower leg is predominantly about assessment of the shafts of the tibia and fibula rather than the joints at either end; however, a systematic approach must still be applied.

The lower leg is another example of a ring structure formed by the tibia, fibula, and proximal and distal tibiofibular joints. Injury to one part often causes a second injury to another.

Whilst it is rare to get a true AP/lateral of both knee and ankle joints on the respective lower leg projection, they can be used to assess for any rotation at a fracture site.

Systematic Approach

Radiographic appearances of the lower leg (Fig. 6.26)

Anteroposterior and lateral projections

Follow the standard approach to the AABCSS in addition to:

Adequacy	• Are both the knee and ankle joints included on the images?
	• Is there overlap if entire anatomy not included on image?
Alignment	• Are the bones of the knee and ankle joints grossly aligned (remember, these are not dedicated projections)?
	• Are the knee and ankle joints grossly AP/lateral to each other dependent on the projection (i.e. are both AP on the AP projection)?
	• Is there any rotation between the knee and ankle?
Bones	• Assess the tibia and fibula in their entirety, trace the cortices, and assess the internal texture
	• Assess any other visible bones at the end of the images:
	• Distal femur
	• Talus
	• Calcaneum
Cartilage (Joint spaces)	• Not dedicated views, difficult to assess joint spaces
	• Is there any gross narrowing/widening (diastasis) of the knee/ankle joints?
	• Is there any gross narrowing/widening (diastasis) of the ankle joint (particularly medially)?
	• Is there any gross widening of the proximal and distal tibiofibular joints?
Soft tissues	• Is there soft tissue swelling?
	• Evidence of lipohaemarthrosis on lateral (if horizontal beam) – see page 158
Significant areas	• In young paediatric patients assess the tibia carefully for subtle lucent lines
	• Assess the distal tibiofibular joint (syndesmosis) for widening
	• Assess the bones at the edge of the images

Fractures/Trauma

Tibia and Fibula Shaft Fractures

(Figs. 6.27 and 6.28)

Fractures to the shaft (diaphysis) of the tibia and fibula are common due to a range of different mechanisms. As the tibia is the weight-bearing bone (the fibula is not), fractures of it are more significant than those of the fibula.

They often occur together, and there are a range of fracture patterns including:
- Transverse, spiral or oblique
- Comminuted: often has a triangular '*butterfly*' fragment
- Segmental: proximal and distal fracture lines leaving a separate central segment

Depending on the complexity and degree of comminution, these fractures might be treated conservatively, or with an intramedullary nail, or external 'Ilizarov frame' fixator. Due to a relatively poor blood supply, these fractures have a relatively high rate of non-union or delayed union, and open fractures are prone to osteomyelitis infection.

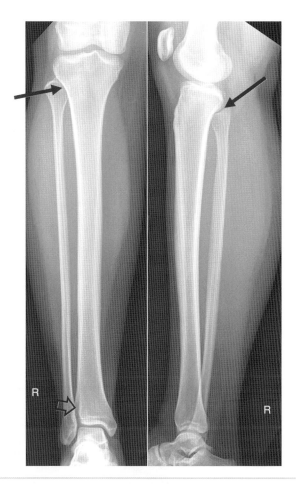

Fig. 6.26 AP and lateral lower leg projections: systematic approach. Adequacy – are both knee and ankle joints included? Is there overlap between the images (if needed)? Alignment – are the knee and ankle joints grossly AP/lateral with each other (i.e. no rotation between them)? Are the bones of the knee and ankle joints grossly aligned? Bones – carefully check ALL of the tibia and fibula; assess the visible distal femur, talus, and calcaneum (and any other visualized bones). Cartilage – difficult to assess joints as not dedicated projections; is there any gross widening/narrowing of the: knee joint, ankle joint (especially medially), proximal (arrow)/distal (hollow arrow) tibiofibular joints? Soft tissues – is there any soft tissue swelling? Evidence of lipohaemarthrosis (if horizontal beam lateral). Significant areas – paediatrics; subtle lucent lines in tibia; distal tibiofibular joint (syndesmosis) for widening (hollow arrow) on AP; assess the bones at the edge of the images. (Source: Bontrager's Textbook of Radiographic Positioning and Related Anatomy, Tenth Edition, 2021.)

Whilst not usually difficult to diagnosis radiographically, it is important to assess the injuries in terms of:

- The fracture pattern/type
- Rotation between the knee and ankle joints
- The presence of shortening (overlapping of the fractured bones)
- Intra-articular extension into the knee or ankle joints and distal tibio-fibular syndesmosis (all may need dedicated imaging)

Fig. 6.27 Segmental tibial and fibula fracture. There are fractures of the proximal and distal shaft of the tibia (arrows) resulting in a 'segment' between them. There is also a fracture of the fibula (hollow arrow). Note the rotation between the AP knee and lateral ankle joints! (Source: Diagnostic Imaging: Musculoskeletal, STATdx © Elsevier.)

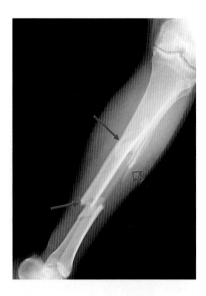

Fig. 6.28 Open tibial and fibula fracture. There are triangular 'butterfly' fragments (arrows) of the mid-tibia and fibula. The overlying bandage artefact suggests this is an open fracture and therefore prone to osteomyelitis. Again, note the rotation between the AP knee and lateral ankle joints on the edge of the image. (Source: Diagnostic Imaging: Musculoskeletal, STATdx © Elsevier.)

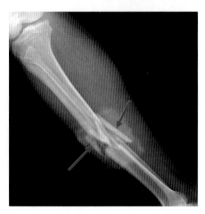

 INSIGHT

As well as having a risk of neurovascular injuries, tibia/fibula fractures also may lead to compartment syndrome. The muscles in the lower leg (and thigh) are found in compartments surrounded by a tough outer fascia. Bleeding within these compartments increases the pressure and reduces blood supply to the muscles and can cause necrosis. As such, it is a significant clinical consideration in lower limb injuries.

Toddler Fracture
(Fig. 6.29)

As the name suggests, this injury is found in young children just starting to learn to walk. The injury occurs either as a result of the new stresses put upon the bone or as a result of a fall whilst the child is still unstable.

As with other stress fractures, radiographic appearances often do not appear for several days after onset of symptoms. Whilst it can occur in other bones in the lower limb, the tibia is by far the most common and classic injury.

Fig. 6.29 Toddler's fracture. A clear lucent spiral fracture line (arrow) is evident on the lateral projection but not the AP. Note the ill-defined nutrient line (curved arrow) on the AP and how its appearance differs from the fracture. (Source: Diagnostic Imaging: Musculoskeletal, STATdx © Elsevier.)

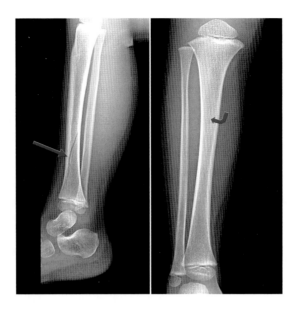

Typical mechanism of injury:
- Fall, often twisting injury
- Repetitive trauma/stress

Clinical presentation:
- Newly walking child; ~1–3 years in age
- Pain, refusal to weight-bear

Appearance:
- May be occult initially, only being visible up to ~10 days after symptoms
- Spiral lucent line in distal shaft/metaphysis of tibia
- May only be evident on one projection
- No displacement
- Be careful not to confuse with nutrient line (see Chapter 2, page 22)

 INSIGHT

Whilst such injuries are well documented within newly walking children, if fractures occur in children in a younger age group, those not yet walking, or without a clear relevant clinical history, then suspected physical abuse should be considered in any lower extremity fracture.

ANKLE

The ankle is one of the most commonly injured joints in the body. It is a complex area to review radiographically, and there are many considerations in terms of different mechanisms which can cause a combination of bone and soft tissue injury. The standard projections when imaging the ankle are the AP mortise and lateral, with lots to consider on each.

Anteroposterior Mortise Projection

This projection is different to a true AP, where the leg would be in the standard anatomical position, but it does not provide a clear visualisation of the ankle joint. Therefore, more commonly, the projection is taken with the leg in slight (approximately 15°) internal rotation to more clearly visualise the ankle joint.

Adequacy (Fig. 6.30)   The purpose of this projection is to gain a clear visualisation of the joint between the talus, lateral malleolus of the fibula, and the medial malleolus and distal articular surface (plafond) of the tibia – the mortise joint.

There is normally a clear and even space all the way around without superimposition of the bones. To achieve this, the foot must be dorsiflexed and the leg sufficiently internally rotated.

As with any joint projection, it should be centred over the joint space and include the skin borders medially and laterally to allow assessment for swelling.

Alignment (Fig. 6.30)   The talar dome should sit within the middle of the mortise joint and articulate with the distal tibial articular surface (called the *plafond* – French for ceiling). The joint surfaces should be parallel and the talus not displaced medially or laterally.

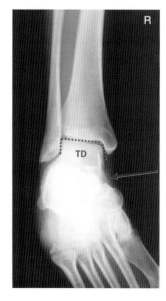

Fig. 6.30 AP mortise projection; adequacy and alignment.
Adequacy – is the mortise joint clear (dotted line)? Alignment – does the talus sit in the middle of the mortise? Does the talar dome (TD) align with the tibial articular surface (top of dotted line)? Are the tarsals in the foot aligned (arrow)? (Source: Bontrager's Handbook of Radiographic Positioning and Techniques, Tenth Edition, 2021.)

Assess the alignment of the other visualised bones with the talus. Dislocations of the tarsals, even very displaced ones, may be overlooked if not assessed.

Bones (Fig. 6.31)

Follow each of the bones carefully around their cortex, looking for subtle steps or interruptions. Look at the internal bone texture for any lucent or sclerotic lines. Follow the:

- *Fibula:* start at the lateral cortex proximally; follow it inferiorly around the lateral malleolus and then superiorly along the medial cortex. Review the internal texture from superior to inferior.
- *Tibia:* similarly start from the point you stop on the fibular and follow the lateral cortex inferiorly, across the plafond, around the medial malleolus, and superiorly along the medial cortex. Review the internal texture from superior to inferior.
- *Talus:* follow the talar dome from lateral to medial. Assess the internal texture for any lucencies, particularly the medial and lateral corners.

Avulsion fractures are common around the tips of the two malleoli, so assess the areas distal to these.

What other bones are visualised is dependent on the projection, but look at them all in turn, especially any metatarsals and the base of 5th metatarsal if included.

In paediatric patients it is important to assess the physeal growth plates for widening.

Fig. 6.31 AP mortise projection; bones.
Assess each bone; follow the cortex and assess internal texture: fibula (F), tibia (Ti), talar dome (TD). Tips of medial and lateral malleolus (arrows) for avulsion fractures. Assess visible bones in foot, including: metatarsals (1–4); base of 5th metatarsal (5). Paediatrics: assess for widening of distal fibula/tibia physeal growth plates – note normal sclerotic remnant of tibial physeal plate on this mature skeleton (curved arrow). (Source: Bontrager's Handbook of Radiographic Positioning and Techniques, Tenth Edition, 2021.)

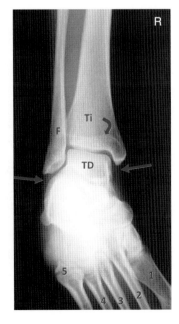

INSIGHT

It is common to see a remnant of the tibial physeal growth plate in mature skeletons as a thin sclerotic line above the joint on both projections, and it should not be mistaken for a fracture.

Cartilage (Fig. 6.32)

Several assessments and measurements related to the ankle joint can be taken (assuming a well-positioned projection):

Mortise joint:
- should be uniform medially, laterally, and superiorly; assess for any widening
- the joint space (in an average adult) should be less than 4 mm; more than 6 mm is suggestive of injury
- look for small intra-articular bone fragments, most commonly from the talus

Distal tibiofibular joint (syndesmosis):
- There is normally overlap between the distal tibia and fibula as the fibula lies posteriorly to the anterior tibial tubercle. A loss of overlap indicates significant injury to this joint.
- The space between the fibula and facet on the tibia, called the syndesmotic space, should normally be 4–6 mm. A measurement in excess of 8 mm is suggestive of injury.
- A sub-optimally positioned mortise can mimic/hide this widening.

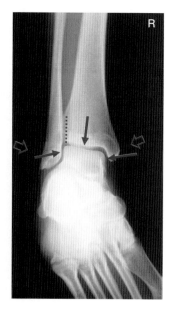

Fig. 6.32 AP mortise projection; cartilage (joints) and soft tissues. Cartilage (joint spaces) – mortise joint: uniform joint space; medially, superiorly, and laterally (arrows); any part of the joint widened – >6 mm? Syndesmosis – is there overlap of the distal tibia and fibula (dotted line)? Is the syndesmotic space widened – >8 mm? Soft tissues – general soft tissue swelling? Swelling over the medial/lateral malleoli (hollow arrows). (Source: Bontrager's Handbook of Radiographic Positioning and Techniques, Tenth Edition, 2021.)

INSIGHT

As part of a ring structure, widening of the medial joint space and/or syndesmosis is normally accompanied by a fracture of the fibula. If there is widening of either without a visible corresponding fracture of the fibula, then it is advised to assess for a proximal fracture using projections of the tibia/fibula (see page 193).

Soft Tissues (Fig. 6.32) Since soft tissue, particularly ligamentous, injury is common in ankle injuries, there is commonly soft tissue swelling to be seen, particularly adjacent to the medial and lateral malleoli, so compare the thickness of the soft tissues.

Focal soft tissue swelling like this is indicative of injury, and whilst it may often be soft tissue, it should be considered enough to warrant further suspicion for bony fracture.

Significant Areas (Fig. 6.33) There are several review areas which must be considered again, even if they have been looked at once:

- *Talar dome:* look within the bone adjacent to the joint surface for any lucencies caused by an avulsed osteochondral fracture (see page 193). In particular, compare the appearance of the medial and lateral corners.
- *Syndesmosis/medial joint space:* is there any widening of the distal tibiofibular or medial ankle joint? If so, is there fracture of the fibula? If there is no visible fibula fracture, then consider tibia/fibular projections.

Fig. 6.33 AP mortise projection; significant areas. Talar dome – lucencies in the medial/lateral corner (arrows)? Tips of medial/lateral malleoli. Syndesmosis/medial joint space – any evidence of widening (curved arrows)? If yes, is there a visible fracture of the fibula proximally (hollow arrow)? Are tibia/fibula projections needed? (Source: Bontrager's Handbook of Radiographic Positioning and Techniques, Tenth Edition, 2021.)

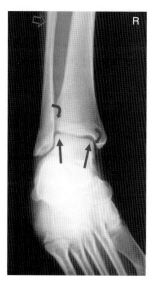

  - *Proximal fibula:* assess for fractures on edge of image, related to the previous point
  - *Tips of malleoli:* look for any subtle fractures distal to the medial and lateral malleolus

Systematic Approach

Radiographic appearances of the ankle, AP mortise projection (Figs. 6.30–6.33)

Anteroposterior mortise projection

Follow the standard approach to the AABCSS in addition to:

Adequacy	• Is the mortise joint clear? • Is the image centered over the ankle joint?
Alignment	• Is the talus centrally aligned with the tibial articular surface? • Are the tarsals of the foot aligned?

Bones	• Assess the bones tibia and fibula in their entirety; trace the cortices and assess the internal texture:
	  • Fibula
	  • Tibia
	  • Talus
	• Tips of medial and lateral malleolus; avulsion fractures?
	• Assess any other visible bones at the end of the images:
	  • Metatarsals
	  • Base of 5th metatarsal
	• Pediatric patients widening of the tibial/fibula physeal growth plates?

Cartilage (Joint spaces)	• Mortise joint:
	  • Check for uniform space; medial, lateral, superior
	  • Is any part of the joint widened (>6 mm)?
	• Syndesmosis:
	  • Overlap between the tibia and fibula?
	  • Is the syndesmotic joint space widened (>8 mm)?

Soft tissues	• Is there soft tissue swelling? • Is there swelling overlying the medial or lateral malleolus?

Significant areas	• Talar dome; check for lucencies or medial/lateral corner
	• Syndesmosis/medial joint space; is it widened?
	  • If yes, is there a fracture of the fibula?
	  • If no fracture, then consider tibia/fibula projections to assess for proximal fracture
	• Proximal fibula fracture on edge of image?
	• Tips of malleoli; any avulsion fracture?

Lateral Projection

The lateral projection may be used to assess both the ankle and calcaneum. For a dedicated lateral calcaneum projection the same systematic approach can be utilised for the visualised portions, though remember, it is not a dedicated projection for the ankle joint and therefore should not be used to assess the joint with certainty.

Adequacy (Fig. 6.34)   There should be a clear joint space between the distal tibia and talar dome. The medial and lateral aspects of the talar dome should be superimposed.

It is important to ensure that the base of 5th metatarsal is included, as a fracture often presents with ankle symptoms and may be caused by injury to the ankle.

Alignment (Fig. 6.34)   Ensure the talar dome articulates with the distal tibial articular surface (plafond) and the lateral malleolus is superimposed over the talar dome.

The tarsal bones should all be aligned:
- Talus with calcaneum inferiorly and navicular anteriorly
- Navicular with cuneiforms anteriorly and cuboid inferiorly
- Calcaneum with talus superiorly and cuboid anteriorly
- Cuneiforms with the metatarsal bases (if included)

Bohler angle:
- Used to assess the integrity of the calcaneum and the presence of compression fracture
- Angle formed between two lines using features of the calcaneum:
  - Between the superior part of the calcaneal tuberosity and the posterior facet
  - Between the posterior facet to the anterior process
- Normally between 20° and 40°, a reduction to <20° suggestive of calcaneal fracture

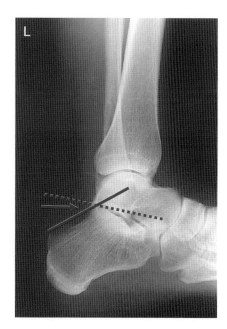

Fig. 6.34 Lateral ankle projection; adequacy and alignment. Adequacy – is the ankle joint space clear? Is the base of 5th metatarsal included? Alignment – is the talar dome aligned with the tibial plafond? Are the tarsals all aligned at their respective joints? Bohler's angle of calcaneum: line drawn from superior aspect of calcaneal tuberosity through posterior facet (solid line); line drawn from anterior process through posterior facet (dotted line); angle between them (arrow) normally 20–40°. (Source: Bontrager's Textbook of Radiographic Positioning and Related Anatomy, Tenth Edition, 2021.)

Bones (Fig. 6.35)

Follow each of the bones carefully around their cortex, looking for subtle steps or interruptions. Look at the internal bone texture for any lucent or sclerotic lines. Follow the:

- *Fibula:* start at the posterior cortex proximally, follow it inferiorly around the lateral malleolus, and then superiorly along the anterior cortex. Review the internal texture from superior to inferior.
- *Tibia:* similarly start from the point you stop on the fibula and follow the posterior cortex inferiorly, across the plafond, and superiorly along the anterior cortex. Review the internal texture from superior to inferior.
- *Talus:* follow the talar dome from its anterior aspect on the head, along the neck and talar dome, and then around the inferior surface. Assess the internal texture for any lucencies, particularly the talar dome and neck.
- *Calcaneum:* start at the anterior process and follow in a similar way to the talus. Inspect the internal texture for lucent line or sclerosis, particularly of the anterior process, the superior articular surface, and the body.

Ensure all visible bones are assessed in the same way in turn, including; navicular, cuboid, cuneiforms, and metatarsals.

Also specifically look for:

- Avulsion fractures on the superior aspect of the foot
- Fracture of the base of 5th metatarsal

Fig. 6.35 Lateral ankle projection; bones. Assess each bone, follow the cortex and assess internal texture: fibula (F), tibia (Ti), talus (Ta), calcaneum (Ca), navicular (N), cuneiforms (Cn), cuboid (Cu). Assess base of 5th metatarsal (arrow). Dorsum of foot for avulsion fractures (hollow arrow). (Source: Bontrager's Textbook of Radiographic Positioning and Related Anatomy, Tenth Edition, 2021.)

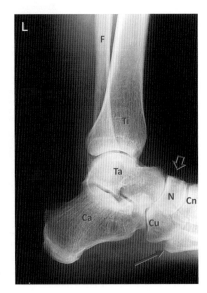

INSIGHT

There are numerous accessory/secondary ossicles found in the foot and ankle (Fig. 6.74), which should not be confused with fracture. One of the most common is the *os trigonum,* which, where present, is found adjacent to the posterior part of the talus. Another is the *os peroneum*, found adjacent to the base of the 5th metatarsal.

Cartilage (Joints)
(Fig. 6.36)

There is relatively minimal consideration of the joints other than assessing each for widening. The ankle joint and subtalar joints should also be assessed for intra-articular bone fragments.

Soft Tissues (Fig. 6.36)

Dorsum of the foot: look for focal soft tissue swelling over the tarsals, often associated with avulsion fractures

Ankle joint effusion (for an example, see Fig. 6.48):
- Normally there is a longitudinal soft tissue plane between the anterior corner of tibia and head of talus
- An effusion, if present, causes displacement of this anteriorly and increased soft tissue opacity in anterior aspect of joint
- Like in the knee or elbow, indicates presence of abnormal fluid in joint

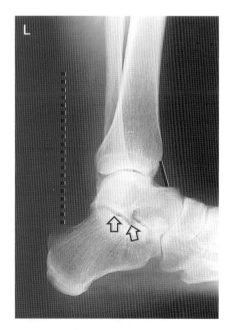

Fig. 6.36 Lateral ankle projection; cartilage and soft tissues.
Cartilage – intra-articular bone fragments in ankle and subtalar (hollow arrows) joints; remaining joints of uniform width. Soft tissues – swelling over dorsum of foot? Bulging of normal fat plane (solid line) with anterior joint opacity to indicate effusion? Achilles tendon: any depression in the posterior soft tissues? Does the Achilles tendon (dotted line) insert in the posterior aspect of the calcaneus? (Source: Bontrager's Textbook of Radiographic Positioning and Related Anatomy, Tenth Edition, 2021.)

Fig. 6.37 Lateral ankle projection; significant areas. Anterior process of calcaneum (solid line); base of 5th metatarsal (arrow); shaft of fibula, edge of image (F); neck of talus (hollow arrow); talar dome (curved arrow). (Source: Bontrager's Textbook of Radiographic Positioning and Related Anatomy, Tenth Edition, 2021.)

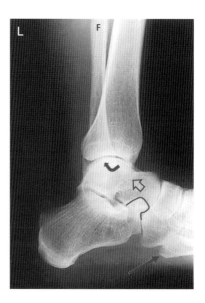

- Following trauma, this is most likely blood (haemarthrosis) and suggestive of injury, though not necessarily fracture. Conversely, a lack of effusion does not rule out injury.

Achilles tendon: whilst not readily visible on radiographs, occasionally rupture may be evident through either a depression in the posterior soft tissues or even evidence of retraction and bunching of the Achilles within the distal calf.

Significant Areas

(Fig. 6.37)

A couple of areas of the lateral ankle projection warrant a specific assessment:

- *Anterior process of calcaneum:* undisplaced fractures may be overlooked
- *Base of 5th metatarsal:* fracture often presents with ankle symptoms and may be caused with injury to the ankle
- *Shaft of fibula:* fractures may be obscured by the tibia, or on the edge of the image
- *Neck of talus:* assess for lucent fracture line
- *Talar dome:* assess for lucency/defect in articular surface which may indicate osteochondral fracture

Systematic Approach **Radiographic appearances of the ankle, lateral projection (Figs. 6.34–6.37)**

Lateral projection

Follow the standard approach to the AABCSS in addition to:

Adequacy	• Is the ankle joint space clear?
	• Is the base of 5th metatarsal included?
Alignment	• Is the talar dome aligned with the tibial articular surface?
	• Are the tarsals of the foot aligned at their respective joints?
	• Are the bases of the metatarsals aligned with the cuneiforms (if included)?
	• Is Bohler's angle of the calcaneum between 20° and 40°?

Bones	• Assess the bones in their entirety, trace the cortices, and assess the internal texture:
	• Fibula
	• Tibia
	• Talus
	• Calcaneum
	• Navicular
	• Cuneiforms
	• Cuboid
	• Metatarsal bases (if included)
	• Assess the base of 5th metatarsal
	• Are there any avulsion fractures along the dorsum of the foot?
Cartilage (Joint spaces)	• Ankle and subtalar joints – any intra-articular bone fragments?
	• Are the joints in the foot normal in width?
Soft tissues	• Is there soft tissue swelling overlying the dorsum of foot?
	• Is there an ankle joint effusion?
	• Achilles tendon:
	• Any significant depression in the posterior ankle soft tissues?
	• Is the Achilles tendon visible and inserting on the posterior calcaneum?
Significant areas	• Anterior process of calcaneum
	• Base of 5th metatarsal
	• Shaft of fibula, superior edge of image
	• Neck of talus
	• Lucencies/defects in talar dome

Fractures/Trauma

There are a multitude of different injury patterns that may occur around the ankle joint, which may involve a combination of bone and soft tissue injuries. The mechanism of injury (what happened to the ankle) can be an important indicator of the types or patterns of injuries that might be visible, or not, on radiographs. The main types of injury can be loosely divided into:

- Inversion and eversion injuries
- Pilon fractures
- Talus dislocation
- Talus fracture
- Calcaneum fracture
- Paediatric Salter-Harris fractures – triplane/Tillaux

Inversion and Eversion Injuries

'Twisting' or 'going over' on the ankle is one of the most common mechanisms of injury and may be a combination of either inversion (medial angulation of the foot) or eversion (lateral angulation of the foot) with rotation.

Picturing the movement of the ankle at the time of injury, and the forces involved, can help to predict the typical injuries that occur. When rotating the ankle, there will be compression forces acting on one side of the ankle and traction forces on the other which often provide sufficient force to cause more than one injury: soft tissue and/or bony.

With such injuries we need to consider three main potential areas for injury due to these mechanisms:

- The medial malleolus and/or deltoid (medial) ligament
- The lateral malleolus/fibula and/or lateral ligament complex
- The talar dome (medial or lateral corner)

These descriptions are a simplified version, as it is a very complex subject! Differences occur, and we also need to consider other areas that may be injured in twisting injuries, such as the base of 5th metatarsal, the anterior process of calcaneum, and the posterior malleolus of the tibia, so a proper satisfaction of search is essential.

Stability of an ankle fracture, and the likely need for surgical management, is particularly related to three aspects which would indicate an unstable fracture:

- Involving both medial and lateral malleoli
- Trimalleolar fractures: the medial, lateral, and posterior malleoli (Fig. 6.42)
- Diastasis (widening) of the syndesmosis (integral to ankle stability)

When considering fractures of the ankle, the Weber classification (Fig. 6.40) is widely used to describe the location of a fibular fracture in relation to the tibial plafond (articular surface) as an indicator of stability and degree of management (i.e. Conservative or surgical).

Weber Classification	Location of Fibula Fracture	Orientation of Fracture	Stability	Typical Mechanism
A	Distal to tibial plafond	Avulsion/transverse	Stable (unless medial malleolus also fractured)	Inversion
B (most common)	At level of tibial plafond	Spiral/oblique	Stable/unstable (dependent on syndesmosis injury)	Eversion
C	Superior to tibial plafond	Transverse/oblique	Unstable (syndesmosis usually ruptured)	Eversion

Inversion Injuries

(Figs. 6.38 and 6.41)

The most common mechanism, inversion injuries, causes medial rotation (adduction) of the ankle joint along with internal rotation (supination) of the foot. Such an injury causes a number of different forces to occur, mainly:

- Traction on the lateral malleolus and lateral collateral ligament complex
- Compression of the medial malleolus by the medial aspect of the talar dome

These forces may lead to a number of typical/common injuries at predicted sites.

- Laterally:
  - Avulsion/transverse/spiral fracture of the lateral malleolus
  - sprain of the lateral ligaments
  - widening of the lateral joint space
- Oblique fracture of the medial malleolus
- Osteochondral injury of the medial aspect of the talar dome

In the adult skeleton a sprain of the lateral ligaments is most common following an inversion injury and, besides lateral soft tissue swelling, there may be no other radiographic findings.

Fig. 6.38 Inversion injuries. A, The talus rotates medially (curved arrow) causing compressive forces medially (green arrow) and traction forces laterally (blue arrow). **B,** Such forces typically result in: spiral/transverse/avulsion fracture of lateral malleolus (LM) OR lateral ligament sprain (arrow); oblique fracture of medial malleolus (MM); lateral joint space widening; osteochondral fracture of medial talar dome (T). Not all may be present. (Source: Bontrager's Handbook of Radiographic Positioning and Techniques, Tenth Edition, 2021.)

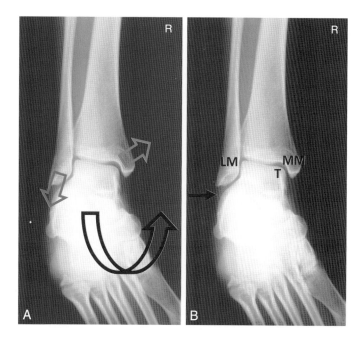

Fig. 6.39 Eversion injuries. A, The talus rotates laterally (curved arrow), causing compressive forces laterally (green arrow) and traction forces medially (blue arrow). **B,** Such forces typically result in: spiral/oblique fracture of lateral malleolus (LM)/fibula shaft (F); diastasis of the syndesmosis (hollow arrow); transverse/avulsion fracture of medial malleolus (MM); OR medial deltoid ligament sprain (arrow); medial joint space widening; osteochondral fracture of lateral talar dome (T). Not all may be present. (Source: Bontrager's Handbook of Radiographic Positioning and Techniques, Tenth Edition, 2021.)

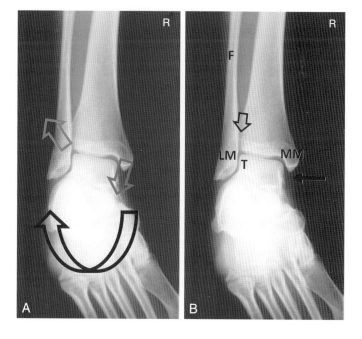

Fig. 6.40 Weber classification of ankle injuries. Predictor of fracture stability in ankle injuries dependent on location of fibula fracture in relation to the tibial plafond and syndesmosis (*). **A,** Fracture distal to tibial plafond/syndesmosis (stable). **B,** Fracture at level of tibial plafond/syndemosis (stable/unstable). **C,** Fracture superior to tibial plafond/syndesmosis (unstable). (Source: McRae's Orthopaedic Trauma and Emergency Fracture Management, Third Edition, 2016.)

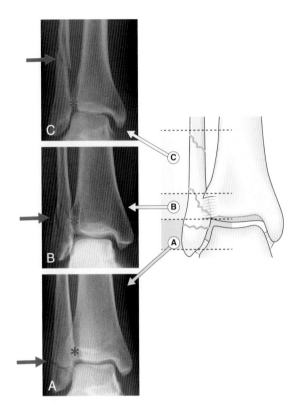

Fig. 6.41 Weber A fracture – inversion injury. Classic appearance of an inversion injury causing a transverse fracture of the lateral malleolus (arrow) and a subtle oblique fracture of the medial malleolus (hollow arrow). There is no joint space widening or lucency within the medial talar dome (curved arrow) to suggest osteochondral fracture. This is a Weber A fracture, as the fibula fracture is inferior to the tibial plafond. (Source: Diagnostic Imaging: Musculoskeletal, STATdx © Elsevier.)

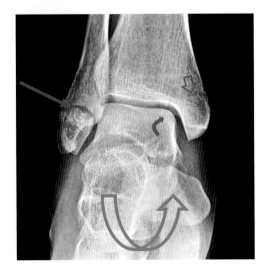

Eversion Injuries

(Figs. 6.39, 6.42–6.44)

Such injuries cause lateral rotation (abduction) of the ankle joint along with external rotation (pronation) of the foot. Such an injury causes a number of different forces to occur which are the opposite to inversion injuries:

- Traction on the medial malleolus and medial deltoid ligament
- Compression of the distal fibula by the lateral aspect of the talar dome

These forces may lead to a number of typical/common injuries at predicted sites.

- Laterally:
  - Oblique/spiral fracture of the fibula (either distally or proximally), and/or
  - Diastasis (widening) of the tibiofibular syndesmosis
- Medially:
  - Transverse/avulsion fracture of the medial malleolus, OR
  - Sprain of the medial deltoid ligament
  - Widening of the medial joint space
- Osteochondral injury of the lateral aspect of the talar dome

Although perhaps less common, eversion injuries are often more significant and complex due to the resultant instability of the ankle that may result.

As well as this general description, there are some specific types of injury which typically occur as a result of inversion/eversion injuries.

Fig. 6.42 Weber B fracture – eversion injury.
A, There is a spiral fracture of the distal fibula (arrow) at the level of the tibial plafond and syndemosis (*) making this a Weber B. There is also a transverse fracture of the medial malleolus (hollow arrow). There is no joint space widening or lucency within the lateral talar dome (curved arrow) to suggest osteochondral fracture. **B,** On the lateral projection, note the vertically orientated fracture of the posterior aspect of the tibia, commonly known as the posterior malleolus. Fractures of the medial, lateral, and posterior malleolus are commonly known as a ***trimalleolar fracture***. (Source: Diagnostic Imaging: Musculoskeletal, STATdx © Elsevier.)

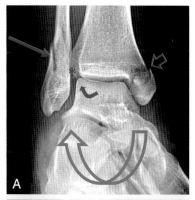

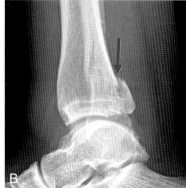

Fig. 6.43 Weber C fracture – eversion injury. There is a comminuted fracture of the fibula (arrow) superior to the syndesmosis (*) which appears widened. There is also a transverse fracture of the medial malleolus (hollow arrow) and lateral displacement of the talus. Note there is a very subtle lucency of the lateral corner of the talar dome (curved arrow) in comparison to the medial corner, suggestive of an osteochondral fracture. This is a very unstable injury. (Source: Diagnostic Imaging: Musculoskeletal, STATdx © Elsevier.)

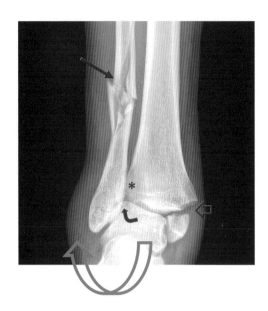

Fig. 6.44 Maisonneuve injury. A, On the initial ankle projections, there is widening of the medial joint space (arrow), and possibly syndemosis (*), without associated visible fibula fracture. **B,** A subsequent image of the lower leg demonstrates an oblique fracture of the proximal fibula (hollow arrow). There will be rupture of the interosseous membrane between the two injuries. (Source: Diagnostic Imaging: Musculoskeletal, STATdx © Elsevier.)

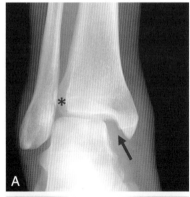

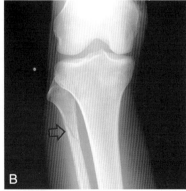

Maisonneuve Fracture (Fig. 6.44)

A variation of the Weber C injury is a significant injury which may well be overlooked. In keeping with the ring theory, an injury of the ankle joint or syndesmosis is normally accompanied by a corresponding fracture of the fibula. Often these are lower and visible on ankle radiographs but sometimes may be higher and nearer the knee with rupture of the interosseous membrane between the fracture and the ankle joint.

When imaging the ankle, if there is no visible fibula fracture in the presence of one or more of the following, then this type of injury must be suspected and typically images of the lower leg performed to assess for a proximal fibula fracture:

- Widening of the medial ankle joint
- Widening of the tibiofibular syndesmosis
- An isolated fracture of the medial malleolus

Typical mechanism of injury:
- Eversion injury; external rotation and pronation of the ankle/foot

Clinical presentation:
- Non-weight-bearing, bone tenderness, swelling to ankle
- Tenderness over fibula fracture (typically distal to knee)
- 'Ottawa positive' on clinical assessment

Appearance:
- Typically no fibula fracture evident on ankle projections
- Presence of one/combination of:
  - Diastasis of syndesmosis/lack of overlap between distal tibia and fibula
  - Widening of medial joint space
  - Isolated transverse fracture of medial malleolus
- Soft tissue swelling; generalised/focal
- Lower leg radiographs demonstrate proximal fracture of fibula

 INSIGHT

The Ottawa ankle rules are clinical signs which indicate high suspicion of fracture and warrant radiographic imaging of the ankle joint. Ankle radiographs are indicated if there is pain in the region of the ankle and one of the following:
- Bone tenderness over posterior aspect of either malleolus
- Bone tenderness over navicular bone or base of 5th metatarsal
- Unable to weight-bear immediately, or in emergency department
There are similar rules related to the knee and foot.

Osteochondral Fracture (Figs. 6.43 and 6.45)

As in other joints such as the elbow and knee, fractures involving bone and the overlying articular cartilage are important to identify, as they can lead to an intra-articular loose body and osteoarthritis.

In the ankle these often occur of the talar dome as a result of inversion/eversion injuries where there is compression against the tibial plafond. They are particularly common in inversion injuries.

Fig. 6.45 Osteochondral fracture of talar dome.
A subtle lucency of the posteromedial aspect of the talar dome (arrows) following an inversion injury is consistent with an osteochondral fracture. In this example there are no other bone injuries evident. (Source: Diagnostic Imaging: Musculoskeletal, STATdx © Elsevier.)

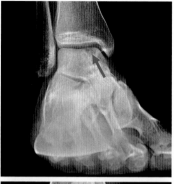

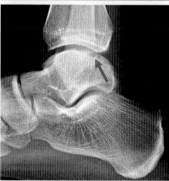

It is important to identify these injuries; they may often be overlooked due to their subtlety or because of other, more significant-appearing injuries.

Typical mechanism of injury:
- Inversion injury (more common than eversion); medial aspect talar dome impacts on tibial plafond

Clinical presentation:
- Non-weight-bearing, bone tenderness, swelling to ankle
- Clicking or locking of ankle

Appearance:
- Often associated with other injuries (e.g. malleolar fractures)
- May appear as:
  - Subtle lucency of corner of talar dome compared to other corner
  - Cortical defect, loss of cortex
  - Small linear intra-articular bone fragment
- Joint effusion possible on lateral

Ankle Dislocation
(Fig. 6.46)

Usually occur as fracture-dislocations in combination with bone fractures; solitary ankle joint dislocations are rare (and not to be confused with talus dislocations discussed below).

Fig. 6.46 Ankle fracture-dislocation. There is loss of alignment of the talar dome (TD) and tibial plafond (Ti) due to a lateral dislocation. There is an oblique fracture of the lateral malleolus (arrows) at the level of the syndesmosis (so Weber B) and an associated avulsion fracture (hollow arrow) from the medial malleolus. This was an eversion-type injury. (Source: Diagnostic Imaging: Musculoskeletal, STATdx © Elsevier.)

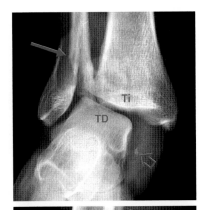

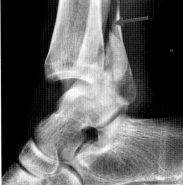

Hallmark is loss of alignment between the talar dome and tibial plafond (distal articular surface). Often subluxed rather than fully dislocated.

Lateral dislocations most common as usually associated with eversion-type injuries.

Other Ankle Injuries

Pilon Fractures
(Fig. 6.47)

Fractures of the distal tibia and tibial plafond. Often as a result of high-energy injuries, they are classically very complex and highly comminuted and often open with significant soft tissue injury. CT is often required for full evaluation prior to management and subsequent osteoarthritis is typical.

Typical mechanism of injury:
- High velocity; talus impacts on tibial plafond (e.g. RTC, fall from height)
- May be low energy (usually less complex); sports injuries, falls

Clinical presentation:
- Non-weight-bearing, bone tenderness, swelling, and bruising to ankle
- May be open
- Possible neurovascular injury

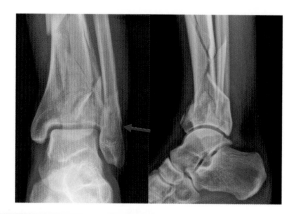

Fig. 6.47 Pilon fracture. There is a highly comminuted fracture of the distal tibia and articular surface (plafond). It is important to look for evidence of open fracture (such as air in the soft tissues), as this is common, though not in this example. There is a less obvious fracture of the fibula (arrow).

Appearance:
- Typically involves a longitudinal fracture of the distal tibia extending into ankle joint
- Most often comminuted, often with multiple fragments
- Fibula fractures and widening of syndesmosis common
- Soft tissue lacerations and air in open fractures
- CT usually required for assessment

Triplane Fracture
(Fig. 6.48)

Similar to a Pilon fracture in that this injury is an intra-articular fracture of the distal tibia and plafond but is only found in adolescents just prior to fusion of the physeal growth plate. As the name suggests, it occurs in three planes/parts:
- Sagittal fracture of the epiphysis
- Transverse 'fracture' through the physeal growth plate
- Coronal fracture of the metaphysis
- This combination of injuries makes it a mixture of Salter-Harris types I, II, and III.

Typical mechanism of injury:
- Eversion/external rotation

Clinical presentation:
- Adolescents (12–15); just prior to fusion of physeal plate
- Non-weight-bearing, pain, swelling to ankle

Appearance:
- Mortice: subtle vertical lucent line through epiphysis into physeal plate (often very subtle)
- Lateral projection: longitudinal/oblique fracture from physeal plate to posterior aspect of tibial metaphysis
- May see widening of physeal growth plate on either projection
- Soft tissue swelling and effusion
- Associated fibula fracture common

Fig. 6.48 Triplane fracture. There is a vertical fracture line of the tibial epiphysis (arrow) on the mortise projection, subtle widening of the anterior and lateral part of the physeal plate (hollow arrows), and a vertical fracture line (curved arrows) from the physeal growth plate to the posterior aspect of the metaphysis. Note elevation of the fat stripe and opacity in the anterior ankle joint (arrowhead) which represents an effusion. (Source: Diagnostic Imaging: Pediatrics, STATdx © Elsevier.)

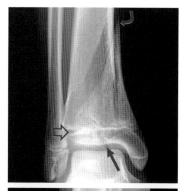
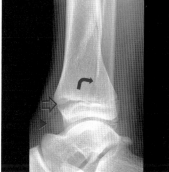

Tillaux Fracture

(Fig. 6.49)

Although a similar injury can occur in adults, causing avulsion of the antero-lateral part of the tibia, most commonly this injury is found in adolescents as a Salter-Harris type III fracture of the lateral part of the tibial epiphysis, adjacent to the syndesmosis.

Although also found in adolescents just prior to closure of the physeal growth plate, unlike the triplane fracture already described, the fracture only occurs in two planes:

- Sagittal fracture of the epiphysis
- Transverse 'fracture' through the physeal growth plate

It occurs laterally within the epiphysis, as this is the last part of the growth plate to fuse (having already done so medially).

Typical mechanism of injury:
- Eversion/external rotation

Clinical presentation:
- Adolescents (12–15); just prior to fusion of physeal plate
- Non-weight-bearing, pain, swelling to ankle

Appearance:
- Mortice:
    - subtle vertical lucent line through lateral part of epiphysis into physeal plate
    - widening of lateral part of the physeal growth plate compared to medial
    - lateral displacement of fragment towards fibula

Fig. 6.49 Tillaux fracture; mortise projection and coronal CT. There is a vertical fracture line (arrows) through the tibial epiphysis and widening of the lateral part of the physeal growth plate (hollow arrows) with lateral displacement. Such a fracture of the epiphysis is known as a Salter-Harris III. Note how the medial aspect of the physeal plate (curved arrow) has nearly fused. (Source: Diagnostic Imaging: Pediatrics, STATdx © Elsevier.)

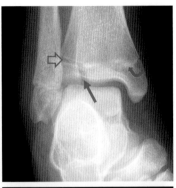

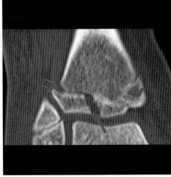

- Soft tissue swelling and effusion
- Associated fibula fracture uncommon

Talus Fractures

(Fig. 6.50)

Besides osteochondral fractures of the talus already discussed, fractures to the rest of the bone may also occur: of the body, neck (most common), and head.

Although often subtle and undisplaced, identification of fractures is important, since the body of the talus shares similarities to the scaphoid and head of femur in relation to its blood supply. Displaced fractures through the neck may lead to osteonecrosis of the body and talar dome and a high risk of osteoarthritis.

These injuries are sometimes given the eponym the 'Aviator's fracture' due to them being seen in the early days of aviation following crashes. CT is widely used to evaluate such injuries, particularly involvement of the subtalar joints.

Avulsion fractures from the superior aspect of the talus head/neck may also be seen.

Typical mechanism of injury:

- Axial loading; foot forcibly dorsiflexed (e.g. in road traffic collision, or plane crash)
- Fall from height

Fig. 6.50 Talus fracture.
There is a lucent fracture line (arrow) extending through the neck of talus towards the subtalar joint (curved arrow) in this undisplaced fracture. Fractures of the neck of talus may lead to osteonecrosis of the body (B) and talar dome. (Source: Diagnostic Imaging: Musculoskeletal, STATdx © Elsevier.)

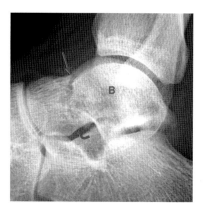

Clinical presentation:
- May be associated with other more significant injuries due to mechanism of injury
- Non-weight-bearing, pain, swelling to ankle

Appearance:
- Best visualised on lateral projection (or oblique foot)
- Lucent line and subtle cortical step within talus
- Assess for intra-articular involvement of the subtalar joints
- May be associated with other fractures/dislocations of the foot and ankle

Talus Dislocation

(Fig. 6.51)

A range of different dislocations related to the talus may occur:
- Subtalar: dislocation of the rest of the foot from the talus at the talocalcaneal and talonavicular joints (the talus remains articulating at the ankle joint)
- Talus dislocation: complete dislocation of the talus from the ankle and subtalar joints (the talus is completely dislocated from the rest of the foot and ankle)

Most occur medially or laterally and are commonly associated with other fractures. There is a high risk of neurovascular injury to the tibial nerve and vessels, so often these dislocations are reduced prior to imaging. As with talus fractures, dislocations may lead to osteonecrosis of the talus.

Typical mechanism of injury:
- High velocity; for example, road traffic collision, fall from height
- Low velocity; sports injuries
- Medial dislocation; inversion on plantarflexed foot
- Lateral dislocation; eversion on dorsiflexed foot

Fig. 6.51 Subtalar dislocation. A, The AP projection demonstrates lateral dislocation (arrow) of the calcaneum (C) and foot in relation to the talus (T). **B,** The lateral projection demonstrates overlap of the talus and calcaneum as a result of the dislocation as well as the clear dislocation of the navicular (N) and head of talus (T) at the talonavicular joint. (Source: Diagnostic Imaging: Musculoskeletal, STATdx © Elsevier.)

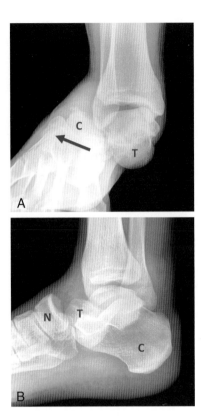

Clinical presentation:
- Non-weight-bearing, pain
- Ankle/foot deformity
- Signs of neurovascular compromise to foot

Appearance:
- Loss of alignment between talus and other bones:
    - Subtalar: between subtalar joint and calcaneum and head of talus and navicular
    - Talus: talus no longer articulating with distal tibia, navicular, or calcaneum
- May be overlooked if not reviewed or due to other fractures
- Assess for associated fractures to talus and other bones during post-reduction imaging

Calcaneal Fractures

Fractures of the calcaneum may be loosely divided into three different main causes:

- Compression fractures
- Avulsion fractures
- Stress fractures

Compression Fractures (Fig. 6.52)

Most commonly seen following a fall from height (sometimes referred to as a lover's fracture for this reason) onto the heel, these injuries are often bilateral. Because of the significant compressive forces involved, which transmit throughout the body, compression fractures of the thoracolumbar spine are also seen in approximately 10% of cases. Fractures to the pelvis, lower limb, and foot may also be found alongside the calcaneal injury.

Most commonly the fracture is comminuted, involves the subtalar joints, and causes flattening of the body, which leads to a reduction in Bohler angle (see page 183). The full extent of the fracture is rarely seen on radiographs, so CT is widely used.

Typical mechanism of injury:

- Axial compression through calcaneum; fall from height most common, road traffic collision

Fig. 6.52 Calcaneal compression fracture. There is a comminuted fracture of the calcaneum with a mixture of sclerotic and lucent areas within the body. The fracture line extends into the subtalar joint (arrows), and Bohler's angle (dotted lines) is greatly reduced. (Source: Diagnostic Imaging: Musculoskeletal, STATdx © Elsevier.)

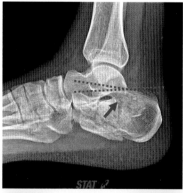

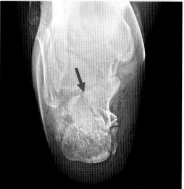

Fig. 6.53 Anterior process calcaneum fracture. There is a lucent line (arrow) through the anterior process of the calcaneum representing an undisplaced fracture. These injuries may be missed unless specifically looked for. (Source: Diagnostic Imaging: Musculoskeletal, STATdx © Elsevier.)

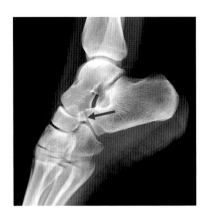

Clinical presentation:
- Significant pain, may mask (or be masked) by other associated injuries
- Bruising to heel
- Other significant fractures and spinal/pelvic injuries may be present

Appearance:
- Best imaged on lateral and axial calcaneum projections
- Reduction of Bohler angle (<20°) on lateral projection
- Combination of lucent/sclerotic fracture lines throughout body
- Assess for intra-articular extension of fracture
- Soft tissue swelling of heel
- Other foot/ankle fractures must be considered

Avulsion Fractures – Anterior Process Fracture (Fig. 6.53)

A number of ligaments and tendons insert on various parts of the calcaneum, such as the Achilles tendon posteriorly, which may cause avulsion fractures.

One of the most commonly overlooked is fracture of the anterior process of the calcaneum, which must always be assessed on both the lateral ankle and oblique foot projections. It may be overlooked as an ankle sprain, but diagnosis and management are essential to prevent subsequent complications.

Typical mechanism of injury:
- Inversion or eversion injury

Clinical presentation:
- Ankle pain and swelling
- Ottawa positive

Appearance:
- Best imaged on lateral ankle/foot and oblique foot projection
- Lucent line through anterior process into calcaneocuboid joint
- Usually minimally displaced

Calcaneal Stress Fracture (Fig. 6.54)

A relatively common site of stress fractures in the lower limb (as well as the distal fibula, proximal tibia, and metatarsals) is the calcaneal tuberosity.

Fig. 6.54 Calcaneal stress fracture. There is an ill-defined band of sclerosis (arrow) within the calcaneum, typical for the appearances of a stress fracture. (Source: Diagnostic Imaging: Musculoskeletal, STATdx © Elsevier.)

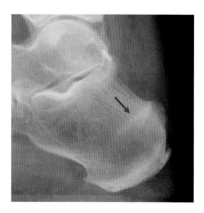

Typical mechanism of injury:
- Stress: repetitive increased force on normal bone (e.g. athletes, jumpers, runners)
- Insufficiency: repetitive normal force on abnormal bone (e.g. in osteoporosis)

Clinical presentation:
- Chronic pain/ache
- Eases with rest

Appearance:
- Initially normal on radiographs, best demonstrated on lateral projection
- Ill-defined band of sclerosis and blurring of trabecular pattern

 INSIGHT

When considering avulsion fractures of the foot and ankle (indeed anywhere in the skeleton), it is important to understand the normal developmental anatomy and ossification centres. One example that causes confusion is the normal secondary ossification centre (apophysis) of the calcaneal tuberosity (Fig. 6.55).

FOOT

Standard projections for the foot are the dorsiplantar (DP) and dorsiplantar oblique (or just oblique). Occasionally a lateral is also performed; many of the review criteria are similar to the lateral ankle.

Adequacy

The DP is not considered an appropriate projection to review the bones of the hindfoot (i.e. the talus and calcaneum) whilst the oblique and lateral does provide somewhat of an overview of this area. As such, it is important that they are included on the image along with the distal phalangeal tufts and all soft tissues.

It is important to ensure that the DP is performed with the foot flat on the image receptor so that there is separation of the metatarsals shafts, but there will be some superimposition of the bases of the 2nd–5th metatarsals.

Fig. 6.55 Normal calcaneal ossification centre. The normal apophysis (arrows) of the calcaneal tuberosity often appears slightly fragmented and sclerotic and should not be confused with fracture. (Source: Diagnostic Imaging: Pediatrics, STATdx © Elsevier.)

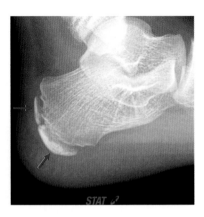

The oblique is turned to provide a sufficiently different view. There should not be superimposition of the metatarsals throughout their length.

Sub-optimal positioning can affect the normal alignment described below and mimic/obscure significant injury.

Alignment

There are some key considerations of the tarsometatarsal (TMT), or Lisfranc, joints that should be appreciated. Appearances as described assume well-positioned images.

Dorsiplantar (Fig. 6.56):

- Normal alignment of the 1st and 2nd metatarsals can be ascertained by:
    - A line along the lateral aspect of the base of 1st metatarsal and the lateral border of the medial cuneiform
    - A line along the medial aspect of the base of the 2nd metatarsal and the medial border of the intermediate cuneiform
- The two lines should be continuous and not be interrupted/have a large deviation
- The two lines should provide a clear space in between them at the 1st intermetatarsal space

Dorsiplantar oblique (Fig. 6.58):

- Normal alignment can be ascertained in three ways:
    - A line along the lateral aspect of the base of the 2nd metatarsal and lateral border of the intermediate cuneiform. A line along the medial aspect of the base of 3rd metatarsal and medial border of the lateral cuneiform. The two lines should be continuous and not be interrupted/have a large deviation. The two lines should provide a clear space in between them at the 2nd intermetatarsal space

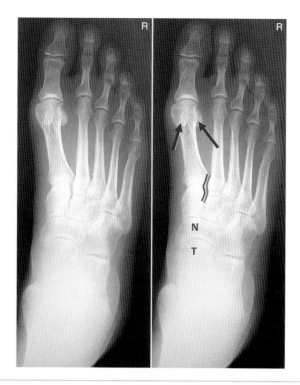

Fig. 6.56 DP foot projection; adequacy, alignment, and bones. Adequacy – note the vertical appearance of the metatarsal shafts; the bases of the 2nd to 5th metatarsals will normally be partially superimposed. Alignment – assess alignment of IP, MTP, and intertarsal joints; alignment of head of talus (T) and navicular (N); continuous lines and space between lines drawn along: lateral aspect base 1st metatarsal and lateral aspect medial cuneiform (red line), medial aspect base 2nd metatarsal and medial aspect intermediate cuneiform (blue line). Bones – each digit in turn; phalanges and metatarsals; tarsals; cuneiforms, cuboid, navicular (N), head of talus (T); any sesamoids; normally two under hallux MTP joint (arrows). (Source: Bontrager's Textbook of Radiographic Positioning and Related Anatomy, Tenth Edition, 2021.)

- Similarly, a line along the lateral aspect of the base of the 3rd metatarsal and lateral border of the lateral cuneiform. A line along the medial aspect of the base of 4th metatarsal and medial border of the cuboid. The two lines should be continuous and not be interrupted/have a large deviation. The two lines should provide a clear space in between them at the 3rd intermetatarsal space
- The articular surfaces of the base of 5th metatarsal and the lateral part of the cuboid should be parallel; the joint should be narrow and equal

Lateral:
- Follow a similar approach to the lateral ankle in relation to Bohler angle and gross alignment of the ankle joint (remember, not a dedicated projection)

Fig. 6.57 DP foot projection; cartilage (joints), soft tissues, and significant areas.
Cartilage – distal and proximal IP joints; MTP joints; clear space between bases 1st/2nd metatarsals and medial/intermediate cuneiforms as per alignment (arrow). Soft tissues – any soft tissue swelling? Significant areas – base of 5th metatarsal (5); bases of 1st to 4th metatarsals (1–4); lateral cortex cuboid (hollow arrow); body of navicular (N). (Source: Bontrager's Textbook of Radiographic Positioning and Related Anatomy, Tenth Edition, 2021.)

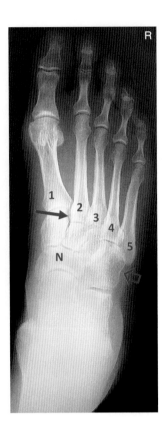

- There should be continuous alignment of the metatarsals and tarsals along the dorsal surface

All other joints between respective bones in the foot should be aligned; be mindful that the phalanges of the toes are often deviated (or hooked) but the joint surfaces should still align.

In particular, assess the alignment of the joint between the head of the talus and navicular on all projections.

Bones

As with the hand, there are a lot of bones to review! Assess each bone in turn: phalanges, metatarsal, and tarsals. Get into a habit of looking at each in turn; for example:

- Start at the distal tuft of the hallux and then assess proximally along each phalanx and metatarsal
- Progress through the 2nd–5th toes in the same way
- Assess the tarsals in a similar way you would the wrist, for example, along the distal row (cuneiforms and cuboid), then the navicular, talus, and calcaneum
- Look at the distal tibia and fibula

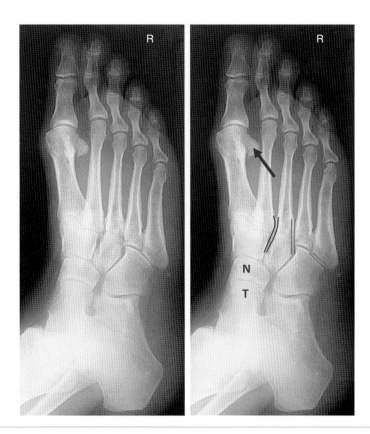

Fig. 6.58 Oblique foot projection; adequacy, alignment, and bones. Adequacy – note the vertical appearance of the metatarsal shafts; the bases of the 2nd-5th metatarsals will normally not be superimposed. Alignment – assess alignment of IP, MTP, and intertarsal joints; alignment of head of talus (T) and navicular (N); continuous lines and space between lines drawn along: lateral aspect base 2nd metatarsal and lateral aspect intermediate cuneiform and medial aspect base 3rd metatarsal and medial aspect lateral cuneiform (red lines); and lateral aspect base 3rd metatarsal and lateral aspect lateral cuneiform and medial aspect base 4th metatarsal and medial cuboid (blue lines); articular surfaces of base of 5th metatarsal and lateral cuboid should be parallel (green lines). Bones – each digit in turn; phalanges and metatarsals; tarsals; cuneiforms, cuboid, navicular (N), head of talus (T); distal tibia/fibula; any sesamoids; normally two under hallux MTP joint (arrow). (Source: Bontrager's Handbook of Radiographic Positioning and Techniques, Tenth Edition, 2021.)

For each bone, follow the cortex looking for steps/interruptions and then the internal trabecular pattern for disruption and lucent/sclerotic lines. Look at the overall shape for any angulations (particularly the metatarsals).

Remember, there will be superimposition of some bones (such as the cuneiforms) on certain projections, so it is important to consider this and assess them on the other projection(s).

The sesamoids of the hallux MTP joint may fracture occasionally, so assess these (there are normally two).

Specific areas to assess:

- The base of all metatarsals (in particular the 5th)
- The anterior process of calcaneum (on oblique and lateral)

- Lateral border of cuboid
- Body of navicular
- The dorsal surface of the tarsals for avulsion fractures (on oblique and lateral)

Cartilage

As with the bones, take time to look at each joint in a similar way; distal/proximal IP and MTP joints of each toe in turn looking for widening or narrowing of each joint (may indicate subluxation/dislocation). Again, angulation of the toes might make this difficult.

As described under alignment there should be a clear space between:

- The base of the 1st/2nd metatarsals and medial/intermediate cuneiform on the DP
- The base of the 2nd/3rd metatarsals and intermediate/lateral cuneiforms, and 3rd/4th metatarsals and lateral cuneiform and cuboid on the oblique
- The lateral aspect of the cuboid and the base of 5th metatarsal on the oblique

Joints between the tarsals should be of fairly equal distance, though the subtalar joint is somewhat wider.

Soft Tissues

Check for general soft tissue swelling on each projection. If there is soft tissue swelling (sign of injury), assess the adjacent area of bone/joint.

On the lateral in particular, dorsal swelling might indicate a small avulsion fracture.

Significant Areas

There are many common fracture areas in the foot, and whilst the previously systematic approach should have identified them, reviewing them again at the end is useful. These include:

- Base of 5th metatarsal
- Anterior process of calcaneum
- Base of 1st–4th metatarsals and joints

Systematic Approach

Radiographic appearances of the foot (Figs. 6.56–6.61)

DP, oblique and lateral projections

Follow the standard approach to the AABCSS in addition to:

Adequacy
- Was the DP performed with the foot flat?
- Is the oblique sufficiently oblique so that the metatarsals are not superimposed?
- Are the tarsals of the hindfoot included?

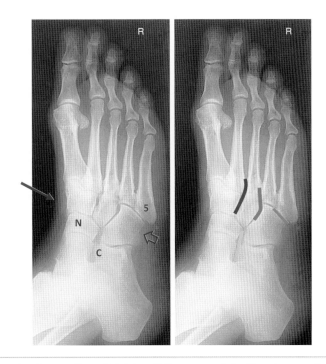

Fig. 6.59 Oblique foot projection; cartilage (joints), soft tissues, and significant areas. Cartilage – distal and proximal IP joints; MTP joints; clear spaces between: bases 2nd/3rd metatarsals and intermediate/lateral cuneiforms as per alignment (red line), bases 3rd/4th metatarsals and lateral cuneiform/cuboid as per alignment (blue line), and lateral articular surface of cuboid and 5th metatarsal (green line); intertarsal joints; note width of normal subtalar joint (yellow line). Soft tissues – any soft tissue swelling, particularly over dorsal surface (arrow)? Significant areas – base of 5th metatarsal (5); bases of 1st to 4th metatarsals; lateral cortex cuboid (hollow arrow); body of navicular (N); anterior process of calcaneum (C). (Source: Bontrager's Handbook of Radiographic Positioning and Techniques, Tenth Edition, 2021.)

Fig. 6.60 Lateral foot projection; alignment and bones. Alignment – assess alignment of IP, MTP, intertarsal, and ankle joints; alignment of head of talus (T) and navicular (N); Bohler's angle (see Fig. 6.34); dorsal alignment of metatarsals and tarsals (dotted line). Bones – each digit in turn; phalanges and metatarsals; tarsals; cuneiforms, cuboid (C), navicular (N), talus (T); distal tibia/fibula; any sesamoids; normally two under hallux MTP joint (arrow). (Source: Bontrager's Textbook of Radiographic Positioning and Related Anatomy, Tenth Edition, 2021.)

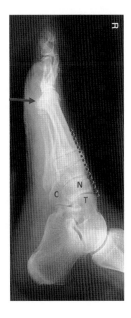

Fig. 6.61 Lateral foot projection; lateral foot projection; cartilage (joints), soft tissues, and significant areas. Cartilage – intertarsal joints; ankle joint. Soft tissues – any soft tissue swelling, particularly over dorsal surface (arrow). Significant areas – base of 5th metatarsal (hollow arrow); cuboid (C); body of navicular (N); anterior process of calcaneum (curved arrow). (Source: Bontrager's Textbook of Radiographic Positioning and Related Anatomy, Tenth Edition, 2021.)

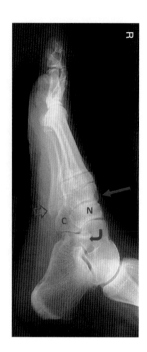

Alignment	• Are all joints grossly aligned (all projections):
	  • Interphalangeal and MTP joints
	  • Intertarsal joints
	  • Head of talus and navicular
	  • Ankle joint
	• *Dorsiplantar projection:*
	  • Alignment and space between base of 1st/2nd metatarsals and medial and intermediate cuneiforms
	• *Oblique projection:*
	  • Alignment and space between base of 2nd/3rd metatarsals and intermediate and lateral cuneiforms
	  • Alignment and space between base of 3rd/4th metatarsals and lateral cuneiform and cuboid
	  • Alignment of articular surfaces of base of 5th metatarsal and lateral part of cuboid
	• *Lateral:*
	  • Bohler angle of calcaneum
	  • Dorsal alignment of metatarsals and tarsals

Bones	• Assess each bone in turn looking for cortical steps/bumps, internal lucent/sclerotic lines, and assess the shape. Follow:
	  • Distal tuft of hallux, phalanx, proximal phalanx, metatarsal
	  • Repeat for 2nd–5th toes
	  • Assess each tarsal turn; distal row (cuneiforms and cuboid), navicular, talus, and calcaneum
	  • Assess distal tibia/fibula
	• Are there any sesamoid bones present? Do they look round, smooth, and adjacent to a joint?

Cartilage (Joint spaces)	• Assess each joint space for narrowing/widening and presence of intra-articular bone fragments • Distal and proximal IP and MTP joints; hallux and other toes • TMT joints (as per alignment) • Intertarsal joints

Soft tissues	• Is there any soft tissue swelling?
	• Is there any swelling over dorsal aspect of foot (oblique/lateral projections)?
Significant areas	• Base of 5th metatarsal
	• Anterior process of calcaneum
	• Base of 1st–4th metatarsals and joints
	• Lateral cortex of cuboid
	• Body of navicular

Fractures/Trauma

 INSIGHT

The Ottawa foot rules are clinical signs which indicate high suspicion of fracture and warrant radiographic imaging of the foot. Foot radiographs are indicated if there is pain in the midfoot (over the tarsals/metatarsals) and one of the following:
• Bone tenderness of the navicular bone or base of 5th metatarsal
• Unable to weight-bear immediately, or in emergency department
There are similar rules related to the knee and ankle.

Navicular Fracture

(Fig. 6.62)

Fractures to the body of the navicular bone are *not common, but they are commonly missed.* They usually occur in the sagittal plane (transverse across the short axis of the bone) and may only be demonstrated on one projection but are prone to avascular necrosis. It is therefore important to include this as part of the systematic approach on all projections.

Avulsion fractures on the dorsal aspect are more common. They should not be confused with two common accessory ossicles, namely *os supranaviculare* and *os tibiale externum*, which occur in the same region (Fig. 6.74).

Typical mechanism of injury:
- Avulsion: inversion or eversion injury
- Body: axial compression between head of talus and cuneiforms (e.g. road traffic collision, fall from height)

Clinical presentation:
- Midfoot pain and swelling
- Ottawa positive
- May be associated with other foot/ankle injuries

Appearance:
- Avulsion:
  - Small linear/triangular fragment
  - Usually over dorsal/medial aspect
  - Sharp, lack a cortical edge; unlike smooth round ossicle
  - Overlying soft tissue swelling
- Body:
  - Subtle lucent line across short axis of bone
  - Often only on one projection
  - May occasionally be comminuted
- Assess for other associated injuries

Fig. 6.62 Navicular fractures. A, There is a subtle avulsion fracture (arrow) of the dorsal aspect of the navicular. There is also an avulsion fracture of the head of talus (hollow arrow). **B,** There is a transverse fracture (curved arrow) across the short axis of the navicular. Such injuries are often only demonstrated on one projection. (Source: Diagnostic Imaging: Musculoskeletal, STATdx © Elsevier.)

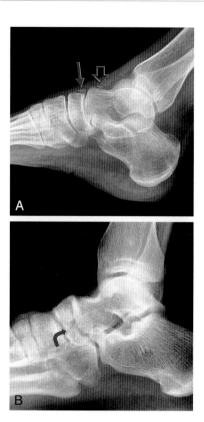

Cuboid Fracture
(Fig. 6.63)

Like navicular fractures, fractures of the cuboid are *not common but commonly missed* on radiographs and are often associated with other injuries of the foot. Fracture lines might be very difficult to identify, so any deformity in its shape or texture should be suspicious.

Typical mechanism of injury:
- Compression; between calcaneum and bases of metatarsals, like a nut in a nutcracker
- May be seen in road traffic collisions or significant eversion-type rotation injuries

Clinical presentation:
- Lateral midfoot pain and swelling
- Ottawa positive
- May be associated with other foot/ankle injuries

Appearance:
- Fracture line not often evident
- Deformity/angulation of lateral cortex
- Sclerosis within body

Fig. 6.63 Cuboid fracture.
There is angulation of the lateral cortex (arrow) and a small fracture fragment (curved arrow) with subtle internal sclerosis (hollow arrow) within the body of the cuboid. (Source: Diagnostic Imaging: Musculoskeletal, STATdx © Elsevier.)

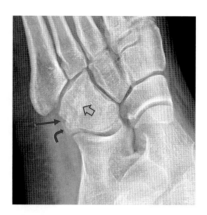

Lisfranc Injuries
(Figs. 6.64–6.66)

Injuries to the tarsometatarsal (TMT), or Lisfranc (after a Napoleonic French surgeon), joints are extremely significant but often overlooked injuries to the midfoot. They may be:

- A ligamentous sprain which demonstrates subtle subluxation of the TMT joints
- A dislocation which demonstrates marked displacement of the TMT joints
- A fracture dislocation of the base of metatarsals

Radiographs may only demonstrate the more severe injuries. A thorough systematic approach to the alignment and evaluation of the bases of the metatarsals is essential to identifying these injuries, which are commonly associated with other fractures, such as to the cuboid. CT and MRI are commonly used to fully assess.

Typical mechanism of injury:
- Forced plantar flexion of foot
- May be high energy (e.g. road traffic collisions)
- May be low energy (e.g. falling off a horse, down a hole, or tripping over clothing)

Clinical presentation:
- Midfoot pain and dorsal swelling
- Ottawa positive
- May be associated with other foot/ankle injuries

Appearance:
- Fractures may be hard to visualise due superimposition of bases of metatarsals and lack of displacement
- Dependent on severity, progressive from sprain to full fracture-dislocation:
    - Often base of 1st metatarsal undisplaced, only 2nd–5th
    - Widening of the proximal 1st intermetatarsal space

Fig. 6.64 Lisfranc injuries. A, Lisfranc sprain; there is rupture of the Lisfranc ligament (hollow arrow) holding the base of metatarsal to the tarsals but no fracture. There may be lateral displacement of the 2nd to 5th metatarsals (arrow). **B,** Lisfranc fracture-dislocation. There is rupture of the Lisfranc ligament (hollow arrow), lateral dislocation of the 2nd to 5th metatarsals (arrow) and a fracture of the base of 2nd metatarsal (curved arrow). (Source: Diagnostic Imaging: Musculoskeletal, STATdx © Elsevier.)

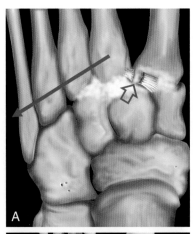

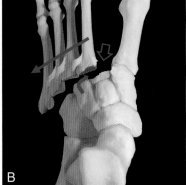

- Loss of alignment at the TMTs on the DP/oblique projection (see page 204)
- Lateral displacement of the metatarsals on the cuneiforms/cuboid
- Dorsal displacement of the metatarsals causes loss of alignment on lateral projection
- Fractures of the bases of metatarsals
- Soft tissue swelling
- May be associated with other foot injuries

Metatarsal Fractures (Fig. 6.67)

More than a third of foot fractures are of the metatarsals, and nearly three-quarters involve the 5th metatarsal. The most common types are: shaft fractures, base of 5th tuberosity avulsion fractures, and stress fractures.

Fig. 6.65 Lisfranc injuries. Two examples of subtle Lisfranc injuries demonstrating only slight loss of alignment and change of the joint space. The oblique projections on both were normal. Sub-optimal positioning can obscure such injuries. **A,** There is loss of alignment/joint space between the 1st metatarsal/medial cuneiform and 2nd metatarsal/intermediate cuneiform. A clear space cannot be drawn between them, and the lines of alignment overlap. **B,** On another example there is widening of the same space as well as a small avulsion fracture fragment (arrow). (Source: Diagnostic Imaging: Musculoskeletal, STATdx © Elsevier.)

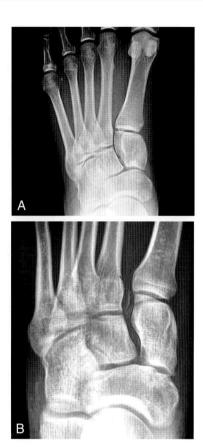

Metatarsal Shaft Fractures (Fig. 6.68)

Common injuries that do not normally cause too much of an issue to identify on radiographs. The 5th metatarsal is the most commonly fractured and the 1st metatarsal the least, and, with the exception of the 5th, fractures typically occur in the distal shaft and neck. Multiple fractures are common.

The 5th metatarsal normally fractures at its tuberosity at the base (discussed separately below) or at its proximal shaft/metaphysis junction, which is known as a *Jones fracture*. This fracture is prone to non-union/delayed union, as this region has a poor blood supply.

Typical mechanism of injury:
- Range of forces; direct blows, crush injuries, eversion/twisting

Clinical presentation:
- Focal pain and swelling – localised tenderness suggestive of fracture and warrants imaging
- Bruising

Appearance:
- Normally transverse/oblique

Fig. 6.66 Lisfranc fracture-dislocation.
A, DP projection; there is widening/loss of alignment between the 1st metatarsal/ medial cuneiform and 2nd metatarsal/intermediate cuneiform with fracture fragment evident (hollow arrow). The 2nd to 5th metatarsals have dislocated laterally (arrow), and there is loss of alignment between the base of 5th metatarsal and cuboid (curved arrow). **B,** Lateral projection; there is subtle loss of alignment between the tarsals and metatarsals (dotted line). Note the overlying soft tissue swelling (hollow arrow). (Source: Diagnostic Imaging: Musculoskeletal, STATdx © Elsevier.)

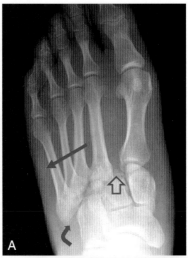

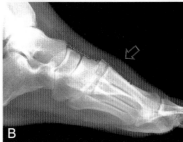

Fig. 6.67 Metatarsal fractures. Location of common metatarsal fractures; the neck/ distal shaft of the 2nd to 4th metatarsals (arrow), proximal shaft/metaphysis of the 5th (hollow arrow) and base of 5th avulsion (curved arrow). (Source: Diagnostic Imaging: Musculoskeletal, STATdx © Elsevier.)

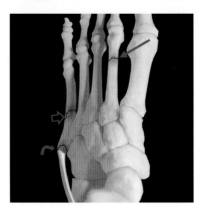

- Most commonly affect shaft or neck of 2nd–4th or proximal shaft/ metaphysis of 5th
- May be minimal displacement
- Sometimes multiple or associated with other fractures
- Soft tissue swelling

Fig. 6.68 Metatarsal shaft fractures. A, Transverse fractures of the neck of 3rd and 4th metatarsals (arrows) with lateral displacement. There is an undisplaced fracture of the shaft of the 2nd metatarsal (hollow arrow). **B,** Transverse fracture of the proximal shaft/metaphysis of the 5th metatarsal. This specific location is referred to as the Jones fracture. (Source: Diagnostic Imaging: Musculoskeletal, STATdx © Elsevier.)

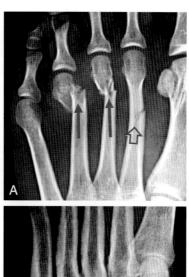

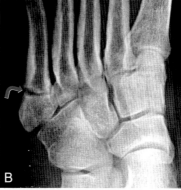

Base of 5th Metatarsal Avulsion Fracture (Figs. 6.69 and 6.70)

Caused by traction of the peroneus brevis tendon, which attaches to the tuberosity at the tip of the base of 5th metatarsal. These injuries are common in a wide range of ankle and foot injuries, and so this is an important review area on both radiographs of the foot and ankle.

Typical mechanism of injury:
- Inversion injuries; avulsion of tuberosity by peroneus brevis tendon

Clinical presentation:
- Focal pain and swelling over base of 5th metatarsal
- Ottawa positive; either ankle or foot

Appearance:
- Transverse/avulsion fracture through base of 5th metatarsal tuberosity
- Normally minimally displaced
- Soft tissue swelling

Fig. 6.69 Base of 5th metatarsal fracture. There is a minimally displaced fracture of the base of 5th metatarsal (arrow). This fracture can be visualised on both foot and lateral ankle projections, so it is a key review area. (Source: Diagnostic Imaging: Musculoskeletal, STATdx © Elsevier.)

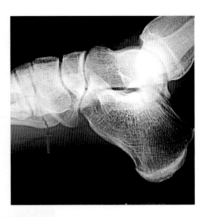

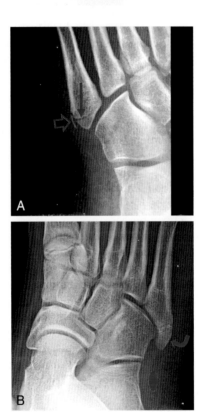

Fig. 6.70 Base of 5th metatarsal fracture and normal variants. A, Apophysis and fracture. There is a minimally displaced transverse fracture of the base of 5th metatarsal tuberosity (arrow). Its horizontal orientation and the fact that it would fit back on indicate it is a fracture. The longitudinal accessory ossification centre of the tuberosity, or apophysis, is a common normal variant seen in immature skeletons (hollow arrow). **B,** Os vesalianum (curved arrow). A normal accessory ossicle found at the base of 5th metatarsal. It can be distinguished from a fracture, as it has a cortical edge all round and its shape makes an abnormally shaped base of 5th metatarsal. Incidentally, another accessory ossicle, Os perineum (oval), is also commonly found more proximally within the peroneus brevis tendon. (Source: Diagnostic Imaging: Musculoskeletal, STATdx © Elsevier.)

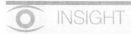

INSIGHT

There are two normal anatomical variants which are sometimes mistaken for fracture of the base of 5th metatarsal (Fig. 6.70):

- Accessory ossification centre (*apophysis*) of the tuberosity: most commonly seen in the immature skeleton but may persist in adulthood. Always orientated longitudinally on lateral aspect of base of 5th metatarsal
- *Os vesalianum:* an accessory ossicle at the base of 5th metatarsal. Is rounded/triangular in shape, has cortical edges, and is too large to fit onto a normal-appearing base of 5th metatarsal

The fracture in contrast to these normal variants always has a transverse/horizontal orientation, is sharp with no cortical edge on the distal part, and would fit back onto the base of 5th metatarsal.

Metatarsal Stress Fracture (Fig. 6.71)

Also more commonly referred to as a *March fracture* due to its association with new soldiers. Most common of the neck and distal shaft. Initially occult on radiographs; periosteal reaction and new bone formation are normally only demonstrated 7–14 days after onset of symptoms.

Typical mechanism of injury:
- Repetitive stress, for example, walking, marching, running
- Stress (fatigue) fracture: abnormal (or new) repetitive stress on normal bone
- Insufficiency fracture: normal stress on abnormal bone (e.g. osteoporosis)

Clinical presentation:
- Focal pain over metatarsal
- Soft tissue swelling
- No acute injury

Appearance:
- Initially normal on radiographs (maybe soft tissue swelling)
- Fuzzy/hazy periosteal reaction around neck of metatarsal after 7–14 days
- Look for very subtle changes in and around cortex
- Faint transverse lucent line
- Excessive hard callous formation may form around fracture
- May form complete fracture if not rested
- Distal shaft/neck more common than proximal metatarsal

Fig. 6.71 Metatarsal stress fracture. Periosteal reaction and new callous formation (arrows) 2 weeks after onset of pain. Initial radiographs were normal. Early findings may be more subtle than this example. (Source: Diagnostic Imaging: Musculoskeletal, STATdx © Elsevier.)

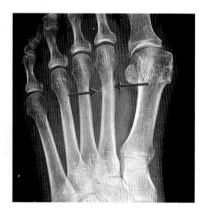

Phalangeal Fractures/ Dislocations (Figs. 6.72 and 6.73)

Although no longer routinely imaged for simple toe fractures, fractures and dislocations of the phalanges are still commonly seen on foot radiographs. A wide range of fracture patterns/dislocations may be seen and a thorough systematic approach of all of the toes is required.

Salter-Harris injuries of the distal phalanges in paediatric patients are common and, as well as open injuries, may be prone to osteomyelitis if they involve the nail bed.

Typical mechanism of injury:
- Range of forces; direct blows (e.g. stubbing toe), crush injuries, hyperflexion/extension

Clinical presentation:
- Focal pain, swelling, and bruising
- May be open

Appearance:
- Range of fracture types:
  - Longitudinal
  - Transverse
  - Oblique
  - Open
  - Salter-Harris involving physeal plates

Fig. 6.72 Phalangeal fracture. An undisplaced longitudinal fracture of the little toes proximal phalanx (arrow), better demonstrated on the DP than the oblique projection. Note fusion of the distal and middle phalanges (hollow arrow) of the little toe, a common normal variant. (Source: Diagnostic Imaging: Musculoskeletal, STATdx © Elsevier.)

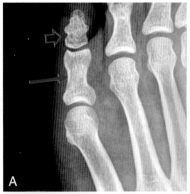

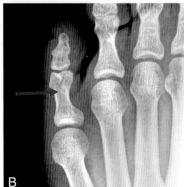

- May have significant/minimal displacement
- Soft tissue swelling
- Assess for soft tissue lacerations and air
- May be mimicked by overlying soft tissue folds/line; soft tissue line will continue past cortex of bone

 INSIGHT

As discussed in Chapter 2, soft tissue/other structures may superimpose bones and mimic fracture lines and cortical steps. This visual illusion is known as the *Mach effect* and is common in the feet where the soft tissues of the toes overlie the phalanges and mimic fracture. It is important to review this area on all projections available and to follow the line; a fracture will stop at the cortex whilst a soft tissue line will often pass beyond the cortex of the bone (Fig. 6.73).

Fig. 6.73 Phalangeal fracture. An intra-articular oblique fracture through the dorsal part of the hallux distal phalanx (arrows). The proximity to the nail bed makes this a possible open fracture and prone to osteomyelitis. Note how overlying soft tissue lines (hollow arrow) caused by the crease of the foot may mimic fracture. (Source: Diagnostic Imaging: Musculoskeletal, STATdx © Elsevier.)

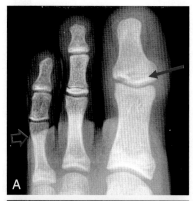

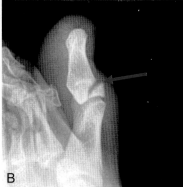

Accessory Ossicles (Fig. 6.74)

As has been alluded to throughout the previous sections, accessory ossicles (either sesamoid bones or accessory ossification centres) are common in the foot and ankle. Their appearance should be sufficient to differentiate from fracture, but an understanding of the common locations can also be very useful.

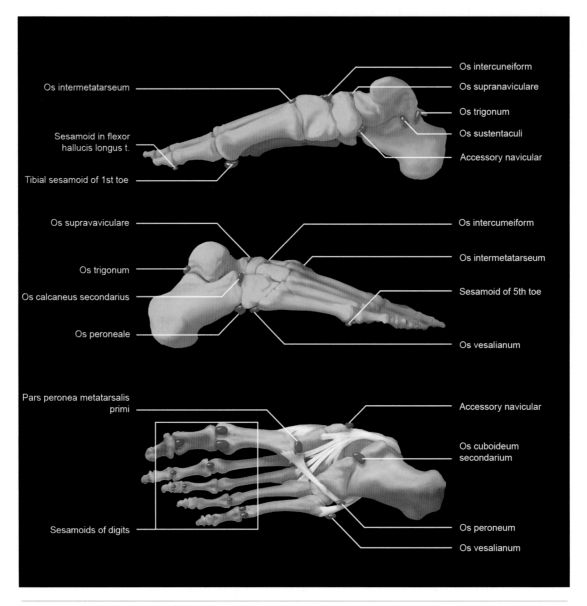

Fig. 6.74 Accessory bones of the foot and ankle. These images demonstrate the location of the most common sesamoid and accessory ossification centres. (Source: Diagnostic Imaging: Musculoskeletal, STATdx © Elsevier.)

PELVIC GIRDLE AND HIP

7

In this chapter we will consider the interpretation of skeletal radiographs of the pelvic girdle, which consists of the two paired innominate (hip) bones and the sacrum, as well as the hip joints.

Whilst the hip joints are included on a pelvis radiograph, we will consider the image evaluation and injuries of the two separately.

PELVIS

Trauma of the pelvis is more commonly now imaged initially using CT in the case of significant trauma, but the anteroposterior pelvis radiograph remains a widely used imaging method. When evaluating the pelvis radiograph, it is important to remember that it does not demonstrate what happened to the bones at the time of injury or visualise soft tissue injury, but there are some rather subtle signs and appearances that can suggest significant injury and trauma.

Adequacy

When imaging the extremities, we usually only image the affected side of the skeleton and so cannot directly compare the appearances against the contralateral (opposite) side, which would be quite useful where features are subtle or equivocal.

With the pelvis, we can use the symmetry of the two sides of the pelvis (and hip joints) to help evaluate the appearances. Rotation of the patient (to left or right) will affect symmetry and therefore appearances between the two sides. It is important therefore to assess the image for rotation by assessing the shape of the bilateral iliac crests and obturator foramen, for example.

Alignment (Figs. 7.1 and 7.2)

The pelvis is a complex structure with each innominate (hip) bone consisting of a number of ridges, spines and processes, depressions, foramen, and fossae. Superimposition of the bone structures results in a number of lines which can be assessed. All should be smooth in contour with no sudden disruptions, interruptions, or changes in shape:

Iliac crests:
- a horizontal line drawn from the superior aspect of one iliac crest should pass through the superior aspect of the opposite iliac crest (assuming the patient is not positioned at an angle to the image receptor)

Main pelvic ring:
- follow the main pelvic ring from the inferior aspect of the right sacroiliac joint, inferiorly along the medial aspect of the ilium, superior aspect of each pubis, superiorly along the left ilium, and across the sacrum
- look for disruptions to the shape of this ring
- remember, the female pelvic ring tends to be more round than the male, which is typically more heart shaped

Fig. 7.1 AP pelvis projection: alignment (1). Iliac crests (red); main pelvic ring (navy blue); obturator foramen (bilateral) (green); Shenton lines (bilateral) (yellow). (Source: Bontrager's Textbook of Radiographic Positioning and Related Anatomy, Tenth Edition, 2021.

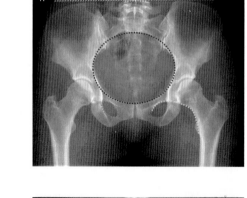

Fig. 7.2 AP pelvis projection: alignment (2). Iliopectineal lines (bilateral) (red); ilioischial lines (bilateral) (navy blue); arcuate lines (bilateral) (green); symphysis pubis (yellow). Note the appearance of Kohler teardrop (arrow). (Source: Bontrager's Textbook of Radiographic Positioning and Related Anatomy, Tenth Edition, 2021.)

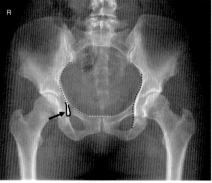

Obturator foramen:
- follow the cortex forming both looking for disruption/steps
- compare the symmetry of the shape of the two

Iliopectineal line:
- used primarily to assess anterior column of acetabulum
- from inferior aspect of the sacroiliac joint, along medial border of ilium and superior aspect of the pubis to the symphysis pubis
- repeat on the opposite side
- disruptions/steps in this line suggest fracture of the anterior column of the acetabulum, or superior pubic ramus

Ilioischial line:
- used primarily to assess posterior column of acetabulum
- follow the medial border of the ilium inferiorly, along the medial border of Kohler teardrop (see below) and along lateral aspect of obturator foramen
- disruption to this line, or displacement of Kohler teardrop, suggests fracture of the posterior column of the acetabulum

Shenton line:
- useful in the evaluation of superior pubic rami and neck of femur [NoF] fractures
- see page 241

Arcuate lines:
- useful to assess for fracture of the sacrum
- follow each of the pairs of sacral foramina; should be smooth and gradual curves
- angulation suggests sacral fracture
- may not be visible/hard to identify due to overlying bowel

Symphysis pubis:
- Superior borders of the pubic rami should be aligned; no step between the two sides
- May be misaligned post-partum or following previous pelvic fracture

 INSIGHT

Kohler's teardrop is an anatomical feature seen on the pelvis radiograph formed by a ridge of bone along the floor of the acetabulum seen end on. It is a useful landmark used in the assessment of pelvic and hip fractures.

Bones (Figs. 7.3 and 7.4)

The bones that comprise the pelvis (the two innominate bones and the sacrum) are complex, and it is worth reviewing their gross anatomy before trying to assess their appearance.

Many of the lines described above for alignment are used to assess fractures by looking for steps, or interruptions in these lines. One method to review the rest of the bones comprehensively is:

Fig. 7.3 AP pelvis projection: bones (1).
Assess symmetry of shape; trace lateral aspect of ilium to acetabulum (red); posterior wall of acetabulum to inferior aspect of pubis (navy blue); lateral margin of sacrum and coccyx (green); repeat for opposite side. (Source: Bontrager's Textbook of Radiographic Positioning and Related Anatomy, Tenth Edition, 2021.)

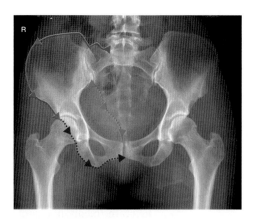

Fig. 7.4 AP pelvis projection: bones (2).
Assess other bones: both proximal femora; inferior lumbar vertebra; note the common sites of avulsion fracture: ASIS (1), AIIS (2), ischial tuberosities (3), lesser trochanters (4). (Source: Bontrager's Textbook of Radiographic Positioning and Related Anatomy, Tenth Edition, 2021.)

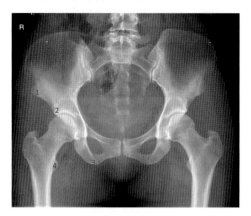

- Look at the overall symmetry of the bones, in particular the iliac crests, sacrum, pubic rami, and proximal femora
- Start at the superior aspect of the right wing of the sacrum and follow the cortex of the iliac crest laterally, then inferiorly along the lateral aspect of the ilium to the acetabulum
- Follow the posterior wall of the acetabulum, then the inferior aspect of the pubis to the symphysis pubis
- Repeat for the left side of the pelvis
- Follow the body of the sacrum on the left and right

Also assess the remainder of the bones:

- Assess the proximal femur on the left and right (see page 242)
- Assess the visualised lower lumbar spine

It is worth remembering that avulsion fractures of the pelvis (see page 239) are commonly found in the following:

- Anterior superior and inferior iliac spines (ASIS/AIIS)
- Ischial tuberosities
- Lesser trochanter of the femur

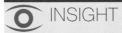 INSIGHT

Secondary ossification centres of the pelvis are some of the last to fuse and should not be confused with avulsion fractures, though actually this is where they do mostly occur! Use symmetry to help differentiate between avulsion fractures and normal ossification centres.

Cartilage (Fig. 7.5)

There are three sets of joints to assess in the pelvis: the sacroiliac joints, hip joints (see page 243), and symphysis pubis.

Sacroiliac joints:

- Difficult to assess accurately on an AP radiograph due to the oblique orientation of the joints (it is rare to see a clear joint space normally) and because of overlying anatomy, particularly bowel
- Can normally see both anterior and posterior aspects of joint separately
- Compare the two joints for symmetry; look for widening or a clear joint space on one side (abnormal) compared to the other. Occasionally abnormal widening may be seen bilaterally

Symphysis pubis:

- Width varies according to age and gender (more mobile in female than male)
- Relatively wide in childhood and prone to degenerative change, so narrower in later years. Typical normal widths:
  - Children ~10 mm
  - Young adults ~6 mm (wider during late pregnancy)
  - Elderly ~3 mm
- Considered abnormal over 10 mm in width at any age

Fig. 7.5 AP pelvis projection: cartilage (joints) and soft tissues. Joints: sacro-iliac joints: note the anterior (blue dotted line) and posterior (red dotted line) parts (normal), assess for symmetry and widening; symphysis pubis (arrow) – less than 10 mm. Soft tissues: obturator fat stripes (green); gluteal fat stripes (yellow); iliopsoas fat stripes (purple). (Source: Bontrager's Textbook of Radiographic Positioning and Related Anatomy, Tenth Edition, 2021.)

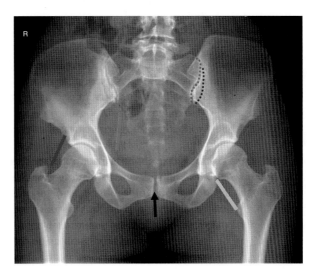

INSIGHT

In keeping with the pelvis being a ring structure, widening (diastasis) of the symphysis pubis post-injury is commonly associated with the widening of a sacroiliac joint(s), and vice versa. Generally, the wider the symphysis, the more unstable the pelvic injury following trauma.

Soft Tissues (Fig. 7.5)

When considering injuries to the pelvis, bone and joint injury is perhaps of less concern than underlying soft tissue injury considering the major organs and structures within the pelvis. This underlying soft tissue injury is rarely visible on radiographs, and is one of the reasons why CT is preferable following major trauma.

However, there are some soft tissue signs on the AP pelvis radiograph which can assist in diagnosing injuries. As with other soft tissue signs, their reliability is often questioned but can raise suspicion of fracture (or other pathology) if present. With the following, assess to see whether they are displaced or obliterated compared to the opposite side:

Obturator fat stripes:
- Longitudinal lines within pelvic ring lateral to sacrum
- Commonly not visualised normally due to overlying bowel gas/faeces

Gluteal fat stripes:
- Medial to neck of femur
- Associated with hip more than pelvic fracture

Iliopsoas fat stripes:
- Lateral to hip joints

Significant Areas

There are a number of areas of the AP pelvis where subtle injuries are found, or pathology missed.

- The acetabulum; assess the area between the femoral head and pelvic ring carefully
- Pubic rami; often subtle or multiple
- The sacrum; body and sacral ala
- Avulsion fractures, particularly ASIS, AIIS, ischial tuberosities, and lesser trochanters

Systematic Approach

Radiographic appearances of the pelvis, AP projection (Figs. 7.1–7.5)

Anteroposterior projection

Follow the standard approach to the AABCSS in addition to:

Adequacy
- Is the patient rotated?

Alignment	• Check alignment and evidence of disruption of:
	  • Iliac crests
	  • Main pelvic ring
	  • Obturator foramen
	  • Iliopectineal lines
	  • Ilioischial lines
	  • Shenton lines
	  • Arcuate lines of sacrum
	  • Symphysis pubis

Bones	• Check symmetry of pelvis for size and shape
	• Start at the right superior sacrum and follow:
	  • Along right iliac crest superiorly and laterally
	  • Inferior along ilium to lateral aspect of acetabulum
	  • Follow posterior part of acetabulum
	  • Along inferior aspect of pubis to symphysis pubis
	  • Trace anterior part of acetabulum
	• Repeat for left side
	• Assess right and left margins and body of sacrum
	• Right and left proximal femora (as per hip checklist, page 245)
	• Lower lumbar vertebra

Cartilage (Joint spaces)	• Sacroiliac joints:
	  • Symmetrical
	  • Assess for abnormal visualisation and widening
	• Symphysis pubis; width less than 10 mm (consider age)
	• Hip joints

Soft tissues	• Check for symmetry and displacement of:
	  • Obturator fat stripes (if visible)
	  • Gluteal fat stripes
	  • Iliopsoas fat stripes

Significant areas	• Both acetabuli
	• Pubic rami; subtle/multiple fractures?
	• Sacrum; body and ala
	• Avulsion fractures:
	  • ASIS
	  • AIIS
	  • Ischial tuberosities
	  • Lesser trochanters
	• Neck of femur

Fractures/Trauma

There are a wide range of injuries which may occur to the pelvis, from the low-energy stable fractures which require minimal management to high-velocity injuries which result in devastating and potentially fatal organ and vascular injuries. It is important to remember that a radiograph does not demonstrate the extent of displacement at the time of injury or the extent of soft tissue injury.

Injuries of the pelvis can be broadly divided into three categories: injuries of the pelvic ring (usually more than one injury), isolated pelvic bone fractures, and acetabular fractures. The main types of injuries that occur include:

- Injuries of the pelvic ring:
  - Anterior compression
  - Lateral compression
  - Vertical shear
- Isolated pelvic fractures:
  - Acetabular fractures
  - Sacral fractures
  - Iliac crest fractures
  - Pubic rami fractures
- Avulsion fractures

 INSIGHT

Considering the pelvis is made of a number of bony rings (the main pelvic ring and the two obturator foramen), high-energy injuries often result in more than one injury: bony and soft tissue. Low-energy injuries can sometimes result in isolated fractures without a second injury to the ring (e.g. acetabular and pubic rami fractures).

Injuries of the Pelvic Ring

Usually a combination of fractures and ligamentous injuries. Pelvic ring may be divided into:

- Anterior – area inferior and anterior to ischial spines (including acetabulum, symphysis pubis, pubic and ischial bones)
- Posterior – areas superior and posterior to ischial spines (including sacroiliac joints and sacrum)

Many injuries are unstable (especially if they involve both anterior and posterior rings), but some are not. CT is usually necessary to evaluate the full extent of injuries and to plan management. They may all have a similar clinical presentation, including:

- Often associated with multiple systemic injuries (e.g. head injury, splenic trauma, other fractures)
- Patient may be unconscious
- Pelvic pain
- Associated neurological signs (e.g. loss of sensation/function)
- Signs of haemorrhage (e.g. hypotension)

 INSIGHT

Ligaments are integral to the strength of the pelvis, particularly those posteriorly around the sacroiliac joints. Damage to these is commonly associated with unstable injuries. Whilst not directly visible on radiographs or CT, widening of the symphysis pubis and/or sacroiliac joints may be an indicator of ligamentous injury.

Anterior Compression (AC) Injuries

(Figs. 7.6, 7.7, and 7.11)

As the name suggests, these injuries are caused by a high-energy force compressing the pelvis from the front to the back. These types of injury often cause diastasis (widening) of the joints of the pelvic ring (symphysis pubis and sacroiliac joints). It is said the pelvis widens like an 'open book', hence the name open book injuries.

They may be associated with associated organ and neurovascular injury, and imaging appearances will often not demonstrate the full degree of displacement at the time of injury. There are three gradings of classification according to the imaging appearances:

Injury Type	Radiographic Appearances	Stability
AC1	Symphysis pubis diastasis <2.5 cm OR bilateral pubic rami fractures SIJ width normal	Stable
AC2	Symphysis pubis diastasis >2.5 cm Anterior SIJ diastasis Posterior SIJ width normal	Relatively stable
AC3	Symphysis pubis diastasis >2.5 cm Anterior and posterior SIJ diastasis OR vertical sacral wing fracture	Unstable

Typical mechanisms of injury:
- High-energy compression or direct blow on the anterior aspect of the pelvis
- Crush injury
- Head-on pedestrian or road traffic collision

Radiographic appearance:
- Dependent on severity
- Often no bony fracture

Fig. 7.6 Anteroposterior compression injury; type 1. There is diastasis (widening) of the symphysis pubis by less than 2.5 cm (arrow) as well as widening of the right anterior SIJ (arrowhead) compared to the normal left (curved arrow). The posterior part of both SIJs is normal. (Source: Diagnostic Imaging: Musculoskeletal, STATdx © Elsevier.)

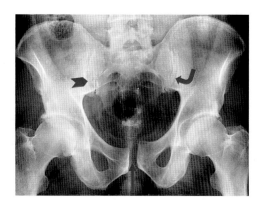

Fig. 7.7 Anteroposterior compression injury; type 2. There is diastasis (widening) of the symphysis pubis by more than 2.5 cm (arrow) as well as widening of the right anterior SIJ (arrowhead) compared to the normal left (curved arrow). It is difficult to assess the posterior part of the SIJs on this projection. Note the difference in appearance of the two sides of the hemipelvis due to lateral rotation of the right side. Also note the normal secondary ossification centres of the iliac crests in this young adult. (Source: Diagnostic Imaging: Musculoskeletal, STATdx © Elsevier.)

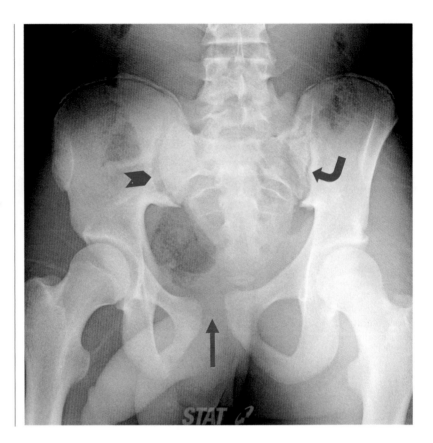

- Look for anterior and posterior injuries
- Anterior:
    - Widening (diastasis) of the symphysis pubis (width important in terms of severity), OR
    - Longitudinal pubic rami fractures; usually bilateral and of both superior and inferior
- Posterior:
    - Widening of the sacroiliac joints; dependent on severity
    - May be unilateral or bilateral
    - Anterior part (more lateral on radiograph, see Fig. 7.5) widened; appears clearer than normal
    - Posterior part (more medial on radiograph) usually normal except in more severe injuries
    - Longitudinal fracture of sacral wing; most severe injuries. May be obscured by bowel. Look for disruption of sacral arcuate lines

Lateral Compression (LC) Injuries

(Fig. 7.8)

Caused by high-energy trauma to the lateral aspect of the pelvis; like in anterior compression injuries, there are three classifications which are a combination of fracture and ligamentous injury.

Fig. 7.8 Lateral compression injury; type 2.
There is a fracture of the left iliac wing (arrow) which extends into the pelvic ring (arrowhead). There are oblique fractures of the superior and inferior left pubic rami (curved arrows). There is disruption of the main pelvic ring (look at the shape compared to Fig. 7.1). (Source: Diagnostic Imaging: Musculoskeletal, STATdx © Elsevier.)

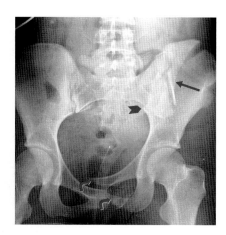

The third type (LC3) is a combination of appearances seen in lateral and anterior compression injuries and is often referred to as a *windswept pelvis* as if a gust of wind (a very strong one) has blown across the pelvis.

Injury Type	Radiographic Appearances	Stability
LC1	Longitudinal impaction fracture of sacrum (on side of injury)	Stable
LC2	Fracture of iliac wing extending into pelvic ring (iliopectineal line)	Relatively stable
	Possible widening of ipsilateral (same) posterior sacroiliac joint	
LC3	Same as LC1 or LC2 on side of injury	Unstable
	Features of AC injury on opposite side (e.g. widening of SIJ and symphysis pubis)	

Typical mechanisms of injury:
- High-energy compression or direct blow on the lateral aspect of the pelvis
- Pedestrian or road traffic collision; hit from side

Radiographic appearance:
- Dependent on severity
- LC1:
    - Vertically orientated impaction fracture of sacrum; increased sclerosis, loss of sacral ala lines
    - May be obscured or very subtle/occult on radiographs
    - Oblique fractures pubic rami fractures possible
- LC2:
    - Fracture of iliac crest/wing which extends into pelvic ring (called 'crescent' fracture)
    - Resultant disruption of iliopectineal line and main pelvic ring
    - Oblique fractures pubic rami fractures possible
- LC3:
    - As per LC1 or LC2
    - Signs of AP compression injury (see page 232) on contralateral (opposite) side of pelvis

Fig. 7.9 Vertical shear injury. There are vertically orientated fractures of the left superior and inferior pubic rami (arrows) and the left sacrum; note disruption of the sacral ala (curved arrow) and the lateral part of the sacrum (*) lying superior to the remainder. There is overall superior displacement of the left hemipelvis compared to the right; note the iliac crest line (dotted line). (Source: Diagnostic Imaging: Musculoskeletal, STATdx © Elsevier.)

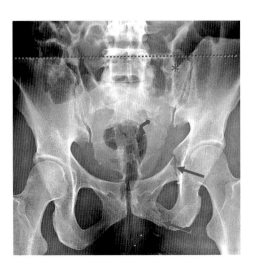

Vertical Shear Injuries (Fig. 7.9)

May be considered the most significant of the pelvic injuries due to higher levels of mortality. They are usually unstable and cause one hemipelvis to be displaced superiorly to the other.

Typical mechanisms of injury:
- High-energy compression; vertical force transmitted through one side of the pelvis
- Typically fall from a height

Radiographic appearance:
- Look for anterior and posterior injuries
- Anterior:
  - Diastasis and misalignment of the symphysis pubis, OR
  - Longitudinal fractures of the pubic rami
- Posterior:
  - Longitudinal fracture of one side of the sacrum, OR
  - Fracture of the iliac wing extending into the pelvic ring (disruption of the iliopectineal line), OR
  - Dislocation of one sacroiliac joint
- Resulting superior displacement of the ipsilateral hemipelvis on the side of the injuries; loss of the iliac crest line (see Fig. 7.1)

Isolated Pelvic Fractures

These injuries may occur in conjunction with injuries to the pelvic ring; however, they can also occur in isolation.

Acetabular Fractures
(Figs. 7.10 and 7.11)

These fractures involve the articular surface of the acetabulum surrounding the femoral head and typically extend into the pelvic ring or obturator foramen. They may occur in isolation or in addition to other pelvic and hip injuries,

Fig. 7.10 Acetabulum fracture. There is a fracture of the posterior wall of the acetabulum (arrow) with a small fracture fragment (arrowhead) and inferior pubic rami fracture curved arrow disrupting the ilioischial line. (Source: Diagnostic Imaging: Musculoskeletal, STATdx © Elsevier.)

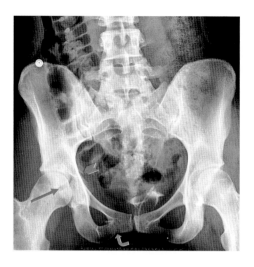

Fig. 7.11 Acetabular fracture and anteroposterior compression injury. There is a transverse fracture of the right acetabulum extending through the posterior wall (arrow), the posterior column disrupting the ilioischial line (curved arrow), and anterior column disrupting the iliopectineal line (arrowhead). Diastasis of the symphysis pubis and left SIJ is consistent with the AP compression injury. (Source: Diagnostic Imaging: Musculoskeletal, STATdx © Elsevier.)

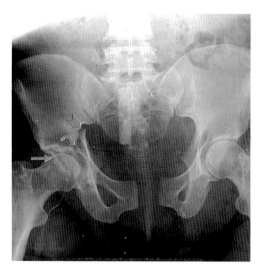

including hip dislocations. There are five main types, involving different parts of the acetabulum:

- Anterior wall – forms the anterior part of the cup surrounding the femoral head; visible overlying medial aspect of femoral head
- Posterior wall – forms the posterior part of the cup surrounding the femoral head; visible overlying the middle of the femoral head (see Fig. 7.3)
- Anterior column – part of innominate (hip) bone between ASIS and symphysis pubis; demonstrated as iliopectineal line
- Posterior column – part of innominate bone between PSIS and inferior pubic ramus; demonstrated as part of ilioischial line
- Transverse – horizontally orientated involving all four of the above

There are usually a combination of the above, and the full extent of the injury is rarely appreciated on an AP radiograph alone; CT is now widely used.

Typical mechanisms of injury:
- High-energy injury; forced compression of femoral head into acetabulum
- Most common in head-on road traffic collisions; dashboard driven into a leg with a flexed hip and knee – usually result in injuries to posterior wall and column
- May occur in patients with osteoporosis in low-energy injury

Clinical presentation:
- Often associated with multiple systemic injuries (e.g. head injury, splenic trauma, other fractures)
- Patient may be unconscious
- Pain over hip joint
- Leg abducted and externally rotated (anterior dislocation) or hip flexed and internally rotated (posterior dislocation)
- Associated neurological signs (e.g. loss of sensation/function), particularly of sciatic nerve

Radiographic appearance:
- Rarely fully assessed on AP pelvis alone
- Assess for fracture line/disruption:
  - Anterior wall of acetabulum
  - Posterior wall of acetabulum
  - Iliopectineal line
  - Ilioischial line
  - Obturator foramen
  - Inferior pubic rami
- Femoral head may be displaced laterally/medially/axially (into pelvic ring)

Sacral Fractures
(Figs. 7.9 and 7.12)

Fractures of the sacrum are notoriously difficult to diagnose on radiographs due to either a lack of displacement or overlying bowel. They may occur in combination with other significant pelvic trauma, in isolation due to injury, or as a stress fracture.

Fig. 7.12 Sacral fracture. There is disruption of the left sacral arcuate lines (arrows) compared to the right (dotted line). These injuries can be extremely subtle! (Source: Diagnostic Imaging: Musculoskeletal, STATdx © Elsevier.)

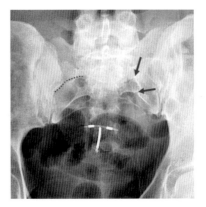

Fractures usually occur vertically orientated through one sacral ala (wing) and are usually associated with high-energy vertical shear injuries or, in isolation, transversely through the entire sacrum. There is a high association (up to half) of neurological injury to the sacral nerves following traumatic fracture.

Typical mechanisms of injury:
- Vertically orientated; high energy, often vertical shear
- Transverse; fall into a seated position

Clinical presentation:
- Often associated with multiple systemic injuries (e.g. head injury, splenic trauma, other fractures)
- Patient may be unconscious
- Pain over sacrum
- Associated neurological signs (e.g. loss of sensation/function)

Radiographic appearance:
- Transverse:
  - Often subtle/occult on radiographs (better assessed on CT)
  - Difficult to assess if minimally displaced
  - Follow cortex of sacrum for step in cortex
  - Disruption in sacral arcuate lines
- Vertical:
  - Disruption of sacral arcuate lines
  - Vertical lucent fracture line
  - Vertical sclerotic band if impaction fracture
  - Superior displacement of lateral part if associated with pelvic ring (vertical shear) injury

Iliac Crest Fracture
(Fig. 7.13)

May occur alone, without further injury to the pelvis or pelvic ring. Also known as a *Duverney* fracture, named after Joseph Duverney in 1751.

Typical mechanisms of injury:
- Direct blow, usually from lateral side

Clinical presentation:
- Pain and bruising

Fig. 7.13 Iliac crest (Duverney) fracture.
Isolated fracture of the iliac crest (arrows). There is no involvement of the acetabulum or pelvic ring; the iliopectineal (arrowhead) and ilioischial lines (curved arrow) are intact. (Source: Diagnostic Imaging: Musculoskeletal, STATdx © Elsevier.)

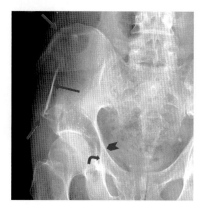

Radiographic appearance:

- Asymmetry between iliac bones
- Cortical step/irregularity of superior/lateral border of iliac crest
- Fracture line within iliac wing
- Iliac crest line might be disrupted
- Normal appearance of other pelvic lines and alignment

Pubic Rami Fractures

(Figs. 7.8–7.10 and 7.14)

Often found in combination with other pelvic injuries but also may occur in isolation either as a single undisplaced pubic rami fracture in patients with osteoporosis or in a '*straddle*' injury where all four pubic rami are fractured (and may be associated with injuries of the genitourinary tract).

The orientation of the fracture gives an indication as to the direction of force: vertically orientated in vertical shear, AP compression, or direct blows; horizontal or oblique in lateral compression.

Typical mechanisms of injury:

- Fall in patients with osteoporosis (single fracture)
- Direct blow to pubic region; 'straddle' injury such as in motorcycle accidents

Clinical presentation:

- Local pain
- May mimic hip fracture

Radiographic appearance:

- Look for cortical step/interruption of pubic rami
- Interruption in iliopectineal, ilioischial, and obturator foramen lines in region of pubic rami
- May be vertical, horizontal, or oblique
- Often undisplaced and subtle
- Satisfaction of search; look for other injuries

Fig. 7.14 Pubic rami fractures. There is a subtle step in the iliopectineal line (arrow) indicating an undisplaced fracture of the superior pubic rami. There is also step in the obturator foramen (arrowhead) and inferior pubic rami (curved arrow) indicating a second fracture. (Source: Diagnostic Imaging: Musculoskeletal, STATdx © Elsevier.)

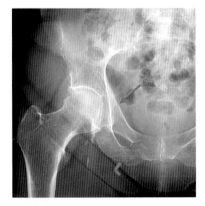

Avulsion Fractures

(Figs. 7.15–7.17)

The apophyses (accessory ossification centres at muscle attachment points) in the pelvis are relatively common sites of avulsion fracture in the pelvis in adolescents once the apophyses have ossified (following puberty) and before they fuse in adults (up to about 25 years). They are rare following fusion of the apophysis except with underlying bone pathology.

Fig. 7.15 Sites of apophysis avulsions.
1 – iliac crest (note normal appearance on Fig. 7.17). 2 – anterior superior iliac spine (ASIS). 3 – anterior inferior iliac spine (AIIS). 4 – ischial tuberosity. 5 – lesser trochanter. 6 – symphysis pubis/inferior pubic rami. (Source: Diagnostic Imaging: Musculoskeletal, STATdx © Elsevier.)

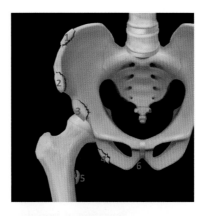

Fig. 7.16 ASIS and AIIS apophysis avulsions.
There are linear bone fragments adjacent to the normal position of the ASIS (arrow) and AIIS (arrowhead) following a kicking injury, in keeping with avulsion fractures. Note the normal iliac crest apophysis (curved arrow). (Source: Diagnostic Imaging: Musculoskeletal, STATdx © Elsevier.)

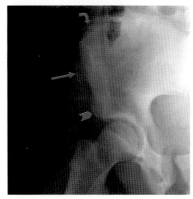

Fig. 7.17 Ischial tuberosity apophysis avulsion fracture. There is a cortical irregularity and rounded bone fragment (arrow) adjacent to the ischial tuberosity in a sprinter with hamstring pain. Again note the normal iliac crest apophysis (curved arrow) not to be confused for fracture. (Source: Diagnostic Imaging: Musculoskeletal, STATdx © Elsevier.)

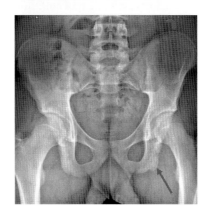

They may be acute with trauma or chronic due to repetitive force on the insertion point. They are often treated conservatively. The sites and muscle attachments where they occur are:

Apophysis	Muscle/Tendon Attachment
Anterior superior iliac spine (ASIS)	Sartorius
Anterior inferior iliac spine (AIIS)	Rectus femoris
Iliac crest	Oblique abdominals
Ischial tuberosity	Hamstrings
Inferior aspect symphysis pubis (inferior pubic rami)	Adductors
Lesser trochanter of femur	Iliopsoas

Typical mechanisms of injury:
- Usually sports; action dependent on muscles involved
- Typically kicking, running, jumping

Clinical presentation:
- Adolescents (~13–25 years)
- Sensation of 'pop' during sports activity
- Localised pain over insertion
- Weakness of affected muscle

Radiographic appearance:
- Bone fragment (varying size) adjacent to the normal site of apophysis
- Loss of symmetry/normal bone contour compared to other side

HIP AND PROXIMAL FEMUR

Anteroposterior Pelvis/Hip

The hip joint and proximal femur are typically imaged using an AP pelvis, which allows assessment of both sides and symmetry between them, but often a dedicated AP hip joint view is also obtained. It is important when reviewing these images that all aspects covered previously on the pelvis are also considered.

Adequacy

The leg when lying supine naturally rotates laterally. This has the effect of shortening the visible neck of femur (NoF) and superimposing the head of femur and greater trochanter over the neck. This greatly limits the ability to visualise fracture.

It is important therefore that the leg is internally rotated slightly when imaging the hip joint in order to elongate the neck of the femur and bring the trochanters into profile to increase the chance of identifying fractures.

Unfortunately, fractures to the NoF, and pain, often leave the leg externally rotated, so we must consider the effect this has on the image and our ability to rule out fracture if internal rotation is not possible.

Alignment (Fig. 7.18)   Besides the lines demonstrated and discussed on the AP pelvis, when considering alignment of the hip joint in trauma, there are a couple of specific aspects to consider:

Shenton line:

- Line following medial cortex of femoral neck and superior border of obturator foramen
- Should be smooth gradual arc/curve
- Assess for interruptions/changes in smooth curve
- Useful in diagnosing femoral neck and superior pubic rami fractures

Femoral neck-shaft angle:

- Lines drawn along long axis of femoral neck and long axis of shaft of femur
- Angle where they bisect normally measures 125–135° (mean of 126° in adults but normally larger in paediatrics and varies according to race)
- Increase/reduction of angle can result from proximal femur fractures (and other pathological conditions)
- Rotation/position of the leg can heavily influence this angle, so consider this when reviewing the image

 INSIGHT

An increase in the femoral neck-shaft angle over 140° is known as *coxa valga* (*coxa* is Latin for hip), where the femoral neck and shaft are more parallel. A reduction in the angle, less than 120°, is referred to as *coxa vara*.

Line of Klein:

- Line drawn along lateral aspect of femoral neck should pass through the lateral aspect of the femoral head epiphysis
- Use symmetry with other hip to compare subtle changes
- Most useful in adolescents to assess for slipped upper femoral epiphysis (SUFE; see page 256)

There are various other angles and measurements which can be taken of the hip when considering hip dysplasia and pathology though these are outside the remit of this text.

Fig. 7.18 AP hip projection: alignment. Shenton's line (navy blue). Line of Klein (red); does it pass through the lateral part of the head (arrow)? Femoral neck-shaft angle (green) between 125° and 135°. (Source: Diagnostic Imaging: Musculoskeletal, STATdx © Elsevier.)

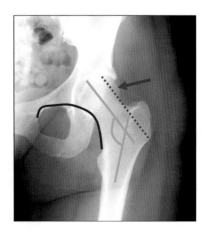

Bones (Figs. 7.19 and 7.20)

Fractures of the proximal femur can be very obvious but often extremely subtle or completely occult (invisible) on radiographs. If both hips are included, then use symmetry to assess size and shape.

Follow the cortex of the lateral shaft of femur, around the greater trochanter, along the femoral neck and head (remember the normal depression of fovea ovale), then down the medial neck of femur, lesser trochanter, and medial shaft of femur. Any change in direction should be smooth without any acute/sharp angles. Pay particular attention to the point where the femoral head and neck meet.

As well as assessing the cortex, the internal trabecular pattern should be used to assess for fracture.

 INSIGHT

The trabecula pattern of a bone follows directions of stress, and larger/more prominent trabeculae follow the direction of most stress. This is related to Wolff law, according to which a bone responds to the forces put upon it (see Chapter 3).

Within the proximal femur there are several 'bands' of trabeculae which are normally visible and can be assessed. The femoral neck-shaft angle means that when weight-bearing, the proximal femur is subject to both tension (pulling) and compression (pushing) forces.

Primary tensile trabeculae:
- Formed by tension forces on the superolateral aspect of the femoral head and neck
- Arc from the fovea ovale on the femoral head to the greater trochanter

Primary compressive trabeculae:
- Formed by compression forces on the head of the femoral head
- Vertical band from the superior aspect of the head to the medial/inferior junction between the head and neck

Secondary compressive trabeculae:
- Formed by compression forces on the proximal femur
- Triangular band from the greater trochanter to the medial femoral neck and lesser trochanter.

Fig. 7.19 AP hip projection: bones. Follow the cortex of the femoral shaft, neck, and head; check the internal bone structure (see Fig. 7.20); assess: greater and lesser trochanters for avulsions, superior and pubic rami, other visualised bones. (Source: Imaging Anatomy: Musculoskeletal, STATdx © Elsevier.)

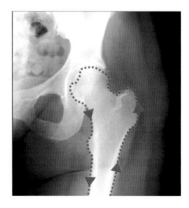

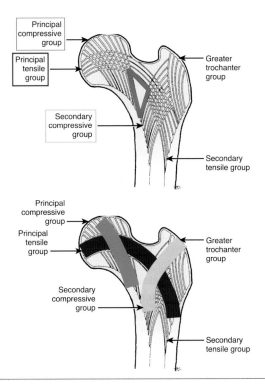

Fig. 7.20 Trabecular pattern, proximal femur. Note the appearances of the normal tensile and compressive trabecular patterns. This is more prominent in some radiographs than others. Ward's triangle (red) lies between the three main groups of trabeculae: primary tensile (blue); primary compressive (green); secondary compressive (yellow). In osteoporotic patients, the primary trabeculae are prominent and Ward's triangle larger but less distinct. (Source: Merrill's Atlas of Radiographic Positioning & Procedures, Fifteenth Edition.)

Between these three groups is a triangular-shaped area which contains minimal trabeculae known as *Ward's triangle*.

When assessing for fractures, look for angulation or disruption of these arcs; sometimes (imagine they are drawn with chalk) it appears as if someone has drawn a finger across and 'smudged' them.

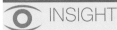 INSIGHT

In patients with osteoporosis (commonly present with neck of femur fractures), smaller trabeculae are resorbed first, leaving the larger primary trabeculae. In this instance, the trabecular patterns described above appear more prominent and Ward's triangle larger and less distinct.

Look for avulsion fractures of the trochanters, as well as fractures in the visualised pelvis (particularly the pubic rami).

Cartilage (Fig. 7.21)

The hip joint space is normally concentric and even between the femoral head and acetabulum (though it is often narrowed in older patients superiorly due to OA).

Fig. 7.21 AP hip projection: cartilage (joints) and soft tissues.
Cartilage – equal hip joint space between femoral head and acetabulum. Femoral head overlapped by anterior rim of acetabulum (red dotted line) and posterior rim of acetabulum (blue dotted line). Soft tissues – gluteal fat stripes (arrow), iliopsoas fat stripes (arrowhead). (Source: Imaging Anatomy: Musculoskeletal, STATdx © Elsevier.)

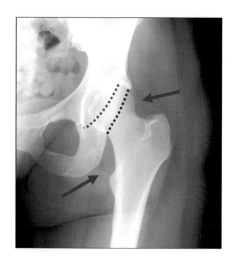

The femoral head should lie between the anterior margin of the acetabulum (medially) and the posterior margin (more lateral and covering more of the head).

Soft Tissues (Fig. 7.21)   As with the pelvis, fat stripes should be assessed (with caution, they are often not reliable) for displacement or if not present:

Gluteal fat stripes:
- Medial to neck of femur
- Associated with proximal femur fracture

Iliopsoas fat stripes:
- Lateral to hip joint

Joint effusions are not reliably assessed on hip radiographs.

Significant Areas   It is important to review the areas where injuries are missed or very subtle, particularly the femoral neck and pubic rami.

If reviewing a dedicated projection of the hip joint, always review the parts of the pelvis which can be visualised (such as the iliopectineal and ilioischial lines).

Systematic Approach

Radiographic appearances of the hip, AP projection (either hip or pelvis projection) (Figs. 7.18–7.21)

Anteroposterior projection

Follow the standard approach to the AABCSS of the pelvis in addition to:

Adequacy
- Is the leg internally rotated; are the trochanters in profile and the neck of femur elongated?

Alignment
- Check alignment and evidence of disruption of:
  - Shenton line
  - Line of Klein
- Is the femoral neck-shaft angle between 125° and 135°?

Bones	• Check symmetry of each femoral head and neck for size and shape (if both included)
	• Trace the femoral shaft, neck, and head from lateral to medial; look for steps or interruptions in the cortex
	• Assess the trabecular patterns for continuity, interruptions, or 'smudging' of:
	  • Primary tensile of the lateral head and neck
	  • Primary compressive, vertical band in the head
	  • Secondary compressive, triangular band across the neck
	• Assess the greater and lesser trochanters for avulsions
	• Assess the visualised portion of the pelvis (e.g. pubic rami)

Cartilage (Joint spaces)	• Hip joint space; equal joint space • Femoral head overlapped by anterior and posterior margins of acetabulum

Soft tissues	• Check for symmetry and displacement of:
	  • Gluteal fat stripes
	  • Iliopsoas fat stripes

Significant areas	• Neck of femur • Both pubic rami • Iliopectineal and ilioischial lines

Lateral Hip

When evaluating the hip for trauma, a secondary projection is always required. In adults this is normally a horizontal beam lateral, which is discussed here. In paediatrics a frog leg lateral projection may be undertaken (the review principles are similar to the AP pelvis).

Adequacy

Often sub-optimal in terms of image quality; it is important to be able to fully assess the head and neck of femur and its articulation in relation to the acetabulum.

Alignment

Like on the AP, there is a normal small angulation between the neck and shaft of femur. The shaft is normally angulated more anteriorly than the neck, though the degree of angulation is dependent on the position of the leg.

Bones

Similar to the AP projection, follow the cortex of the shaft, neck, and head of femur. Assess the internal texture for lucent/sclerotic fracture lines. Consider the sub-capital (junction of the head and neck) region carefully.

Assess both trochanters and ischial tuberosity (posterior to head of femur) for avulsion fracture.

Cartilage

The joint space cannot be accurately assessed; ensure the femoral head is central within the acetabulum and not dislocated anteriorly or posteriorly.

Soft Tissues

There is very little to consider in terms of the soft tissue structures.

Significant Areas

Review the neck of femur for very subtle fractures.

Systematic Approach

Radiographic appearances of the hip, lateral projection (Fig. 7.22)

Horizontal beam lateral projection

Follow the standard approach to the AABCSS in addition to:

Adequacy	• Can the femoral head and acetabulum be visualised?
Alignment	• Is there a slight anterior angulation of the shaft in relation to the neck?
Bones	• Trace the femoral shaft, neck, and head from anterior to posterior; look for steps or interruptions in the cortex • Assess internal texture for lucent/sclerotic fracture lines or disruption to the trabecular pattern • Assess the greater and lesser trochanter • Assess the ischial tuberosity for avulsion fractures
Cartilage (Joint spaces)	• Hip joint space; does the femoral head lie within the acetabulum?
Soft tissues	• Check soft tissues generally
Significant areas	• Neck of femur, especially junction between head and neck

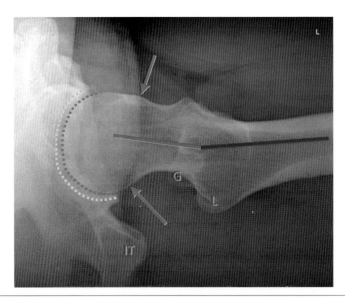

Fig. 7.22 Lateral hip: systematic approach. Adequacy – can the femoral head and acetabulum be visualised? Alignment – slight anterior angulation between femoral neck (red line) and shaft (blue line). Bones – trace the cortex of the femoral shaft, neck, and head; anteriorly and posteriorly; assess for avulsion fractures of the greater (G) and lesser (L) trochanters; assess the ischial tuberosity (IT) for avulsion fractures. Cartilage – does the femoral head (green dotted line) lie central within the acetabulum (orange dotted line)? Soft tissues – is there any soft tissue swelling? Significant areas – assess the neck of femur, especially at the junction of the head and neck (arrows). (Source: Bontrager's Textbook of Radiographic Positioning and Related Anatomy, Tenth Edition, 2021.)

Fractures/Trauma

Fractures and dislocations of the proximal femur and hip can be loosely divided into:
- Fractures of the proximal femur:
  - Head
  - Neck
  - Trochanteric region
  - Sub-trochanteric region
- Hip joint dislocation

Before considering the injuries, it is important to consider some key anatomic features of the proximal femur. The proximal femur is divided into four regions (Fig. 7.23):
- The head: rounded, covered by articular cartilage
- The neck: narrowed portion which is further divided into:
  - Sub-capital; where the head and neck join
  - Cervical (or mid/transcervical); main part of the neck
  - Basicervical; where the neck meets the trochanteric region
- Trochanteric: area between the greater and lesser trochanters
- Sub-trochanteric: the proximal 5 cm region of the shaft below the lesser trochanter

The hip joint capsule covers the head and neck regions, inserting on the femur at the basicervical region. Fractures of the head and neck are classed as *intracapsular*, and fractures of the trochanteric and sub-trochanteric regions are classed as *extracapsular* (Fig. 7.24).

The arterial blood supply for the head comes predominantly from the circumflex branches of the femoral artery which enter distally in the trochanteric region and then pass proximally through the neck and into the head (Fig. 7.25).

Fig. 7.23 Regions of the proximal femur.
1 – head;
2 – neck (specifically cervical part of neck);
3 – trochanteric region;
4 – subtrochanteric region;
5 – shaft.
Subcapital part of neck (red line). Basicervical part of neck (blue line). (Source: Bontrager's Textbook of Radiographic Positioning and Related Anatomy, Tenth Edition, 2021.)

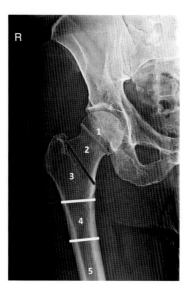

Fig. 7.24 Proximal femur fractures. Can be intracapsular (head and neck) or extracapsular (trochanteric and subtrochanteric regions). (Source: McRae's Orthopaedic Trauma and Emergency Fracture Management, Third Edition, 2016.)

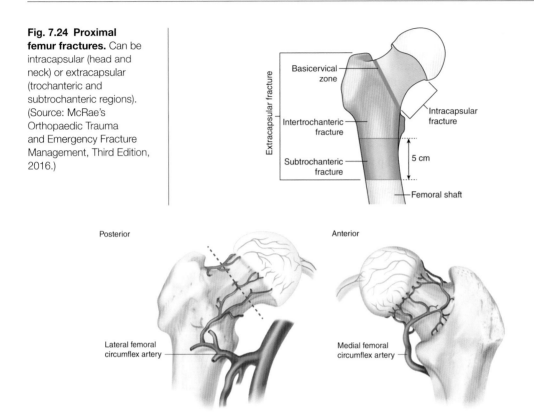

Fig. 7.25 Blood supply of the proximal femur. The large majority of the blood supply to the femoral head comes distally, via the neck. Fractures through the neck (dotted line) can disrupt this supply and cause osteonecrosis of the head. (Source: Fractures of the Proximal Femur: Improving Outcomes, 2011.)

In a similar principle to that of the scaphoid (see Chapter 4, page 90), fractures through the neck, especially if displaced, may disrupt this blood supply and lead to osteonecrosis of the head.

This is seen predominantly in fractures of the neck; fractures of the trochanteric and sub-trochanteric regions (due to the nature of their own blood supply) do not normally result in osteonecrosis. This is an important factor in prognosis and management of the fracture.

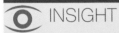 INSIGHT

Displaced fractures through the neck of femur are typically managed with a hemiarthroplasty (replacement of the femoral head) due to the likelihood of osteonecrosis. Fractures of the trochanteric/sub-trochanteric regions are typically treated with screws, plates, and nails (the femoral head is not replaced).

Femoral Head Fracture (Fig. 7.26)

Also known as osteochondral fracture (because it involves bone and articular cartilage) or capital (head) fracture. Much less common than other proximal femur fractures, almost always associated with hip dislocations. May be prone to osteonecrosis of the fracture fragment and osteoarthritis.

Typical mechanisms of injury:
- High-velocity injuries; road traffic collisions
- Same as for hip dislocations

Clinical presentation:
- Hip pain
- Reduced range of movement

Radiographic appearance:
- Often associated with dislocation of hip and possible acetabular fracture
- Often subtle; small linear/crescent-shaped bone fragment adjacent to femoral head
- May see lucency in femoral head (represents donor site from fracture)
- May present as lucent line across femoral head

Neck of Femur (NoF) Fractures (Figs. 7.28–7.30)

Common in elderly and osteoporotic patients as an example of a fragility fracture. Associated with high levels of morbidity and mortality in older patients, and so are treated with urgency. These are types of intracapsular fractures which may occur in the sub-capital, cervical, or basicervical regions (Fig. 7.24).

May be displaced and prone to osteonecrosis, or very subtle/occult on radiographic imaging. Follow-up imaging (MRI/CT) is required if suspicion of fracture persists despite normal (or uncertain) radiographs.

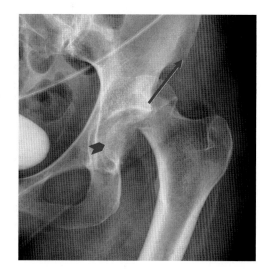

Fig. 7.26 Femoral head fracture and posterior dislocation. There is a fracture through the femoral head (arrowhead) which remains articulating with the acetabulum. The remaining part of the head and femur is dislocated posteriorly (arrow). Internal rotation of the leg (with the greater trochanter in profile) is common with posterior dislocation, but a lateral is needed to confirm the direction of displacement. (Source: Diagnostic Imaging: Musculoskeletal, STATdx © Elsevier.)

Typical mechanisms of injury:
- Commonly low velocity; falls from standing
- May be associated with high-velocity injuries, such as road traffic collision in younger patients

Clinical presentation:
- Usually elderly/osteoporotic patients; may present with other fragility fractures (e.g. Colles, neck of humerus, vertebral)
- Hip pain and bruising
- Reduced range of movement
- Leg shorted and externally rotated

Radiographic appearance:
- Can occur at sub-capital, cervical, or basicervical aspect
- May be very subtle; cortical step/angulation (especially lateral aspect of neck) with disruption or 'smudging' of primary tensile and compressive trabecular pattern
- May be complete fracture with displacement
- Obliteration/displacement of gluteal and iliopsoas fat stripes
- Garden classification (Fig. 7.27) useful to consider radiographic features:

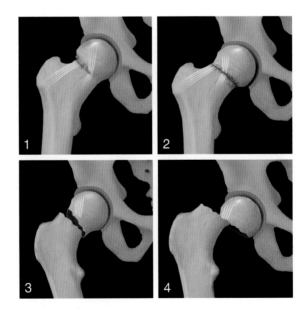

Fig. 7.27 Garden classification of neck of femur (NoF) fractures.
Type I – incomplete, mild valgus angle, step on lateral cortex; type II – complete but undisplaced; type III – complete, minimally displaced, varus angulation (reduction in femoral neck-shaft angle); type IV – complete, displaced. (Source: Diagnostic Imaging: Musculoskeletal, STATdx © Elsevier.)

Garden Classification	Description/Radiographic Findings	Chance of Osteonecrosis for Head
I	Incomplete impaction fracture to lateral part of neck. Slight valgus angulation (increase in femoral neck-shaft angle) but no displacement. Disruption to primary trabeculae	Low
II	Complete fracture through neck, no displacement. Disruption to primary trabeculae	Low
III	Complete fracture through neck. Minimal displacement, varus angulation (reduction in femoral neck-shaft angle; <120°)	High
IV	Complete fracture through neck. Displacement, usually lateral, of distal part on neck	High

Garden I and II fractures may be treated with screw fixation; type III and IV often require hemiarthroplasty due to high risk of osteonecrosis.

Fig. 7.28 Neck of femur fracture; Garden type II. Undisplaced fracture of the subcapital neck of femur. Cortical steps laterally (arrow) and medially (arrowhead) demonstrated it is complete. A subtle area of sclerosis (curved arrow) indicates subtle impaction and 'smudging' of the trabecular pattern. (Source: Diagnostic Imaging: Musculoskeletal, STATdx © Elsevier.)

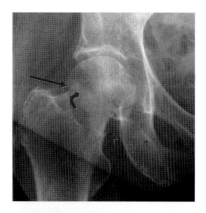

Fig. 7.29 Neck of femur fracture; Garden type III. Minimally displaced complete fracture of the midcervical neck of femur (arrow) with varus (medial) angulation of the shaft – note the reduction in the femoral neck-shaft angle. (Source: Diagnostic Imaging: Musculoskeletal, STATdx © Elsevier.)

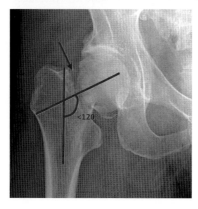

Fig. 7.30 Undisplaced neck of femur fracture.
A very subtle band of sclerosis (arrows) – 'smudging' of the trabecular pattern – demonstrates a very subtle undisplaced midcervical NoF fracture. There is no cortical, step and the iliopsoas (arrowhead) and gluteal fat stripes (curved arrow) are undisplaced. Similar appearances may be evident in a stress fracture and as a result of osteophytes in degenerative disease. (Source: Diagnostic Imaging: Musculoskeletal, STATdx © Elsevier.)

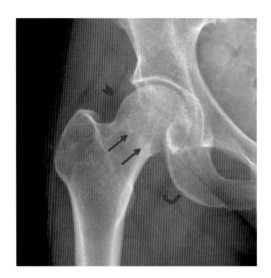

Stress Fracture of Neck of Femur (Fig. 7.30)

Found in both young athletes (stress fracture) and patients with osteoporosis (insufficiency fracture) and can appear similar to an undisplaced NoF fracture. Will become a complete fracture if not treated (usually conservatively).

Typical mechanisms of injury:
- Repetitive low-energy trauma; running, jumping
- Abnormal stress on normal bone; stress fracture
- Normal stress on abnormal bone; insufficiency fracture

Clinical presentation:
- Young athletes or elderly/osteoporotic (or other metabolic bone disease)
- Hip pain
- No acute trauma

Radiographic appearance:
- Horizontal band of sclerosis, 'smudging' of trabeculae, across neck of femur
- Possible loss/displacement of gluteal and iliopsoas fat stripes
- If fracture is complete, as per other NoF fractures

 INSIGHT

It is not uncommon for osteoarthritis of the hip to cause osteophyte (bone spur) formation around the sub-capital region of the neck of femur. This 'ring of osteophytes' can cause a sclerotic appearance similar to an undisplaced neck of femur or stress fracture. Normally osteophytes can be seen on the medial and lateral aspect helping to make the diagnosis (Fig. 7.31). Of course, there may be a fracture present too!!

Fig. 7.31 Ring osteophytes. There is subtle sclerosis of the medial aspect of the neck (arrows). An osteophyte on the lateral (arrowhead) and medial (curved arrow) aspect indicates this appearance is due to a ring of osteophytes rather than fracture. A lateral projection would also demonstrate osteophytes anterior and posteriorly, helping to rule out fracture. (Source: Diagnostic Imaging: Musculoskeletal, STATdx © Elsevier.)

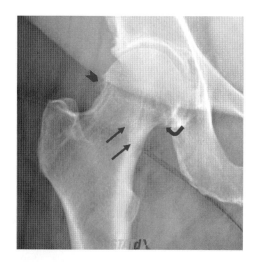

Fig. 7.32 Intertrochanteric fracture part classification. A, two-part; fracture line running between greater and lesser trochanter (may also run in opposite direction between trochanters). **B,** three-part; additional fracture of the greater or lesser (arrow) trochanter. **C,** four-part; additional fractures of both greater and lesser trochanters. (Source: Diagnostic Imaging: Musculoskeletal, STATdx © Elsevier.)

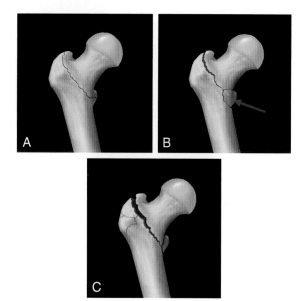

Intertrochanteric Fractures (Figs. 7.32–7.33)

Similar to neck of fractures, intertrochanteric fractures are a common fragility fracture found in older (typically the most elderly) and osteoporotic patients. Intertrochanteric injuries are an extracapsular range of fractures occurring in the region between the basicervical part of the neck superiorly and the inferior part of the lesser trochanter.

Fig. 7.33 Four-part intertrochanteric fracture; AP (A) and lateral (B) projections.
There is a fracture (arrow) between the trochanters causing varus (medial) angulation – the femoral neck-shaft angle is <120°. A separate small fracture of the greater trochanter (arrowhead) and lesser trochanter (curved arrow) makes this a four-part fracture. (Source: Diagnostic Imaging: Musculoskeletal, STATdx © Elsevier.)

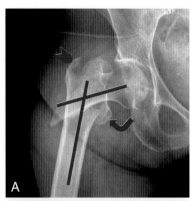

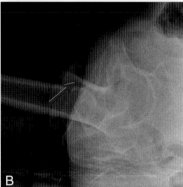

Often more displaced and obvious than neck of femur fractures and typically cause a varus angulation (femur neck-shaft angle <120°), they may be simply classified by the number of fragments (Fig. 7.32):

- Two-part: single fracture line along the intertrochanteric ridge between the greater and lesser trochanter
- Three-part: same as two-part but with separate fracture of either lesser or greater trochanter
- Four-part: fractures along intertrochanteric ridge with separate fractures of greater and lesser trochanters

They do not normally cause osteonecrosis, as they occur distal to the circumflex arteries and are typically treated with internal fixation (such as a dynamic hip screw – DHS) and have a better prognosis than NoF fractures.

Typical mechanisms of injury:
- Commonly low velocity; falls from standing
- May be associated with high-velocity injuries, such as road traffic collision, in younger patients

Clinical presentation:
- Usually elderly/osteoporotic patients; may present with other fragility fractures (e.g. Colles, neck of humerus, vertebral)
- Hip pain and bruising

- Reduced range of movement
- Leg shortened and externally rotated

Radiographic appearance:
- Usually displaced fractures
- Assess for number of parts; 2-,3-, 4-part
- Most commonly cause varus (medial angulation femur neck-shaft angle <120°) though may be valgus
- Isolated avulsion fractures of the greater or lesser trochanters can also occur

Sub-Trochanteric Fractures

Occur within the femoral shaft less than 5 cm inferior to the lesser trochanter. Below this they are classed as femoral shaft fractures but otherwise are practically identical (see Chapter 6, page 151). Such injuries usually require intramedullary nail for treatment.

Typical mechanisms of injury:
- Low velocity: falls from standing in the elderly/osteoporotic/underlying pathology
- High velocity: for example, road traffic collisions

Clinical presentation:
- Elderly/osteoporotic patients: less commonly than neck of femur/intertrochanteric fractures
- Young adults: need to consider other injury if significant mechanism of injury
- Hip pain and bruising
- Deformity if displaced

Radiographic appearance:
- Usually obvious
- Occur within 5 cm inferior to lesser trochanter
- May be transverse, oblique, or comminuted
- May be displaced/undisplaced

Hip Dislocations (Figs. 7.26 and 7.34)

In contrast to those seen in the glenohumeral joint of the shoulder, the majority of hip dislocations (over 90%) are posterior, and less than 10% are anterior. May be associated with fractures to the femoral head (either pre- or post-reduction) and fractures to the pelvic ring and acetabulum.

Typical mechanisms of injury:
- High energy
- Posterior: most commonly road traffic collision – 'dashboard injury' – head of femur in flexed hip pushed posteriorly.
- Anterior: direct blow from behind

Clinical presentation:
- Young adults (fractures more common in elderly)
- Hip pain and deformity, leg shortened and rotated:
  - External rotation – anterior dislocation
  - Internal rotation – posterior dislocation

Fig. 7.34 Anterior hip dislocation. The head of femur is dislocated superiorly (arrow) from the acetabulum (dotted line) and overlying the iliac bone. External rotation of the leg (with the lesser trochanter in profile, arrowhead) is common with anterior dislocation, but a lateral is needed to confirm the direction of displacement. A small bone fragment (curved arrow) may be from the femoral head or acetabulum, and CT is most likely required to assess. (Source: Diagnostic Imaging: Musculoskeletal, STATdx © Elsevier.)

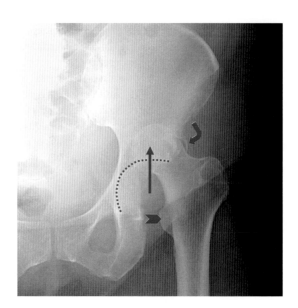

- Reduced range of movement
- May be associated with other significant injuries

Radiographic appearance:
- Loss of congruity of femoral head with acetabulum; anterior/posterior rim no longer superimposed on head of femur
- Loss of Shenton line
- Posterior:
    - femur usually displaced superiorly and laterally
    - leg internally rotated; greater trochanter in profile, lesser trochanter hidden
- Anterior:
    - femur either displaces inferiorly and medially (overlying ischium), or
    - superiorly overlying iliac bone
    - leg externally rotated; lesser trochanter in profile
- Need lateral projection to confirm direction
- Assess for fractures of femoral head, acetabulum, and pubic rami; assess iliopectineal, ilioischial, and obturator foramen lines

Slipped Upper Femoral Epiphysis (Figs. 7.35 and 7.36)
Slipped upper (or capital) femoral epiphysis (SUFE) is a fracture of the physeal growth plate of the proximal femur between the head and neck. The head of the femur 'slips' off the neck posteriorly and medially.

Only occurring in adolescents during growth spurts up until fusion of the physeal plate, it is a type of Salter-Harris 1 injury.

Fig. 7.35 Slipped upper femoral epiphysis (SUFE). Salter-Harris 1 fracture of the physeal growth plate (arrow) causes the femoral head epiphysis to 'slip' posteriorly and medially (curved arrow). (Source: Diagnostic Imaging: Pediatrics, STATdx © Elsevier.)

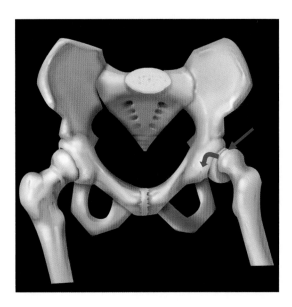

Fig. 7.36 Slipped upper femoral epiphysis (SUFE) right hip. On the AP projection (A), the head of femur on the right appears slightly smaller, and the physeal growth plate (arrows) slightly wider than the left. The frog-leg projection (B) demonstrates the medial and posterior displacement of the femoral head (curved arrow) more clearly. Note the difference in how the line of Klein (dotted line) appears in relation to the head on the left and right hips. (Source: Diagnostic Imaging: Pediatrics, STATdx © Elsevier.)

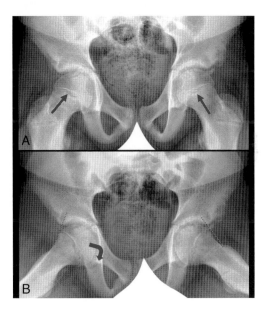

Although normally chronic, it may be acute or following trauma. It is usually unilateral but can be bilateral in approximately a third of cases. It is best imaged using a frog-leg lateral pelvis projection (if possible due to pain), and comparing symmetry between the two hips is very helpful.

Typical mechanisms of injury:

- May occur following trauma; for example, sports injury
- Most commonly chronic

Clinical presentation:
- Twice as common in males than in females; males present later
- Presents following puberty up until fusion of physeal plates; most common 11–14 years
- Obesity increases risk
- Gradual onset hip/thigh pain; may suddenly increase
- Reduced range of movement

Radiographic appearance:
- Depends on degree of displacement; symmetry between hips helpful
- Frog-leg projection more sensitive than AP
- Early; mild widening and irregularity of physeal growth plate
- Later:
  - affected epiphysis shorter than contralateral side
  - line of Klein does not intersect head of femur (or asymmetry with other hip)
  - Shenton line disrupted
  - Head of femur displaced posteriorly and medially

Peri-prosthetic Fractures/Dislocations

Hip prostheses such as total hip replacements, hemiarthroplasties, and other metal fixations are usually stronger than the bone in which they lie. Therefore bones are more prone to fracture than the prosthesis, particularly in the older patient. Typically fractures occur around the tip of the prosthesis where the metal meets the bone.

Dislocations of hip replacements can also occur.

SPINE

8

The spine is a complex structure formed by a collection of irregularly shaped bones. It is important that you have a good understanding of the anatomical features present and how these articulate in order to appreciate their appearance on radiographic images. As with any other axial skeletal anatomy, key principles when considering the radiographic image are symmetry, alignment, and shapes.

CERVICAL SPINE

For all projections check the cortical margins of each bone. This is more complex with the spine due to the numerous features and articulations present causing overlying shadows.

Check for disruption of the cortical and trabecular bone patterns.

Review the bones for any changes in bone density.

 INSIGHT

Due to the irregular shape of the vertebra, there are numerous cortical margins present representing a variety of anatomical features, for example, pedicles and spinous processes. It is important that you are able to recognise these various features and associate them with individual vertebrae.

Lateral

Adequacy

Name, date, marker are the starting point for assessing any image.

Ensure all seven cervical vertebrae are present and the 1st thoracic vertebra is included.

Ensure that all anatomical features are present on the image.

Alignment

Anterior Vertebral Line

This line is located at the anterior aspects of the vertebral bodies and should be a smooth uninterrupted line. This line is represented as the blue line on Fig. 8.1.

Posterior Vertebral Line

This line is located at the posterior aspects of the vertebral bodies and should be a smooth uninterrupted line. This line is also referred to as George's line. This line is represented as the orange line on Fig. 8.1.

Spinolaminar Line

This line is formed at the fusion of the two laminar processes with the spinous process and is located at the anterior aspect of the spinous processes. This line is represented as the red line on Fig. 8.1.

These three lines should all follow a normal curve lordosis representing the secondary curvature of the cervical spine. The normal curvature of the cervical spine is between 20° and 40°.

 INSIGHT

The spinal cord is located between the posterior vertebral line and the spinolaminar line.

Spinous Process Line

This line is used to trace the tips of the spinous process at the posterior aspect of the spinous process. This line is represented as the green line on Fig. 8.1.

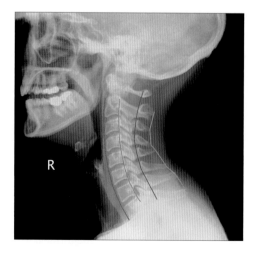

Fig. 8.1 Lateral cervical spine lines. Anterior vertebral line (blue), posterior vertebral line (orange), spinolaminar line (red), spinous process line (green). (Source: Gray's Anatomy: The Anatomical Basis of Clinical Practice, Forty-Second Edition, 2021.)

Fig. 8.2 Lateral cervical spine shapes and appearances. Harris ring of 2nd cervical vertebra (blue), outline of odontoid process (red), vertebral bodies (green), soft tissue (orange). (Source: Gray's Anatomy: The Anatomical Basis of Clinical Practice, Forty-Second Edition, 2021.)

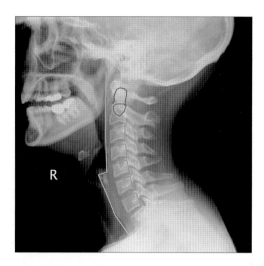

Fig. 8.2 Lateral cervical spine shapes and appearances. Harris ring of 2nd cervical vertebra (blue), outline of odontoid process (red), vertebral bodies (green), soft tissue (orange). (Source: Gray's Anatomy: The Anatomical Basis of Clinical Practice, Forty-Second Edition, 2021.)

Bones

Review the cortical and trabecular patterns of bones. There are numerous bones, so ensure you follow the outline of each individual bone.

The vertebral bodies below the 2nd cervical vertebra should have a uniform oblong shape, as demonstrated by the green outlines on Fig. 8.2.

Odontoid Process (Dens/Peg)

Trace the line from the second body of the cervical vertebra around the odontoid process to note and disruption to the line, as demonstrated by the red line in Fig. 8.2.

Harris Ring

At the 2nd cervical vertebra a ring is noted, as demonstrated by the blue ring on Fig. 8.2. This ring can be incomplete inferiorly. Any disruption to the other aspects of this ring would be suggestive of an odontoid process fracture.

Cartilage

The height of the disc spaces between the vertebral bodies should be approximately equal in height, as demonstrated by the blue shapes in Fig. 8.3.

The facet joints spaces should be uniform; as demonstrated by the green lines on Fig. 8.3 look for any disruption. Please note that if the image is not a true lateral, this can be difficult to assess.

The joint space between the anterior aspect of the odontoid process and the posterior aspect of the anterior arch of the 1st cervical vertebra (pre-dental space) should be no wider than 3 mm in adults and 5 mm in children, as demonstrated by the red line on Fig. 8.3.

Soft Tissue

It is important that the soft tissue is observed in front of the anterior spinal line. Soft tissue thickness anterior to cervical vertebral bodies of those at the level of and above the 4th cervical vertebra should be approximately 33% of the width of vertebral body. The thickness of soft tissue at the level of and below the 4th cervical vertebrae should be approximately 100% of the vertebral bodies, as demonstrated by the orange line in Fig. 8.2. Any increase in size of the soft tissue could indicate injury, due to a haematoma.

Fig. 8.3 Lateral cervical spine lines. Intervertebral disc spaces (blue), joint space between the anterior aspect of the odontoid process and the posterior aspect of the anterior arch of the 1st cervical vertebra (red), facet joint (green). (Source: Gray's Anatomy: The Anatomical Basis of Clinical Practice, Forty-Second Edition, 2021.)

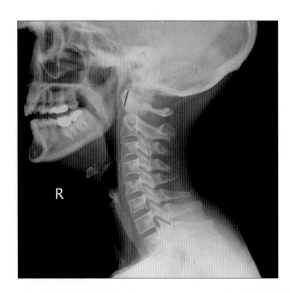

 INSIGHT

The increase in soft tissue size below cervical vertebra 4 is due to the commencement of the oesophagus below this level.

Once you have reviewed the cervical spine, review other anatomical features present, which include the mandible and the base of skull.

Significant Areas

Ensure that the 1st thoracic vertebra is included on the image. Shoulders can obstruct visualisation of the 1st thoracic vertebra. It is suggested that the lateral projection is taken on expiration to aid the lowering of the shoulders.

Noting any disruption to the lines and soft tissue is essential.

Artefacts

Assess whether there are any artefacts present on the image that may affect the interpretation of the image.

Systematic Approach

Lateral view of the cervical spine

Follow the standard approach to the AABCSS in addition to:

Adequacy	• Ensure all anatomy is included • Ensure that the image is lateral
Alignment	• Use lines and follow these to note any disruption to one or more lines
Bones	• Review the cortical and trabecular patterns of bones following the lines. • Review for uniformity of the vertebral bodies below 2nd cervical vertebra.
Cartilage (Joint spaces)	• The vertebral disc height should be approximately equal. • Facet joints should be uniform. • Assess the joint space between the anterior arch and the odontoid peg.

Soft tissues	•	Note any soft tissue swelling of the pre-vertebral soft tissue (the soft tissue is wider below the 4th cervical vertebra).
Significant areas	•	All aspects of the cervical spine can be injured; as such, it is essential to evaluate all the areas identified thoroughly. The lateral cervical spine image will demonstrate most injuries in this region.

Anteroposterior

 INSIGHT

When checking for symmetry in anteroposterior projection, first check the technical quality of the image to ensure that the patient is not rotated. Rotation of the patient will result in loss of symmetry.

Adequacy	Ensure that the cervical spine from the 3rd to the 7th vertebra is included, as well as the upper aspect of the thoracic vertebrae.
	Superimposition of the mandible on the inferior aspect of the occipital bone. This obscures the visualisation of the 1st and 2nd cervical vertebrae.
	The lateral margins of cervical spine need to be included
Alignment	**Spinous Process**
	The spinous process should form a central line Fig. 8.4B. The distance between the spinous processes should be fairly uniform; there should not be any that are 50% wider than the one superior or inferior.
Encompasses Pedicles and Transverse Processes	**Pedicles**
	The pedicles form two straight lines on either side of the spinous process towards the lateral margins of the cervical bodies (Fig. 8.4B).
	Transverse Processes
	Form two straight lines at the lateral aspect of the cervical vertebrae (Fig. 8.4B).
Bones	Review the cortical and trabecular patterns of each individual bone for any disruption. The vertebral bodies should be of an even height (Fig. 8.4C).
Cartilage	The superior and inferior adjacent end plates of the vertebral bodies should be parallel to each other, creating an even space (Fig. 8.4C). Towards the lateral aspects of the vertebral bodies, the end plates are angled, which reflects the uncinate processes (Fig. 8.4C).
Soft Tissues	Assess for any disruption of soft tissue. This could be due to emphysema or an apical pneumothorax may be visible.
Significant Areas	The lines described under alignment heading follow the significant areas where injuries are noted.

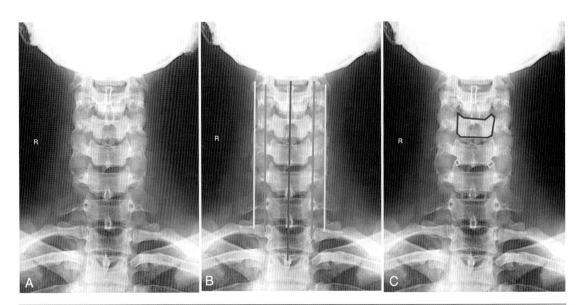

Fig. 8.4 Anteroposterior cervical spine. **A,** anteroposterior view of the cervical spine. **B,** spinous process line (red line), pedicles (bilateral green lines), transverses processes (bilateral yellow lines). **C,** red outline represents a vertebral body. Green outline represents the disc space and the yellow outlines represent the bilateral uncovertebral joints. (Source: Merrill's Atlas of Radiographic Positioning & Procedures, Fifteenth Edition, 2023.)

Systematic Approach

Anteroposterior view of the cervical spine

Follow the standard approach to the AABCSS in addition to:

Adequacy	• Assess the image for rotation.
	• Ensure all anatomy is included.
	• Ensure that the inferior aspect of the mandible and occiput are superimposed.
Alignment	• Use lines and follow these, noting any disruption.
Bones	• Review the cortical and trabecular patterns of bones following the lines.
	• Review for uniformity of the vertebral bodies below 2nd cervical vertebra.
	• The space between the spinous processes should be fairly even.
	• Assess other bones present, for example, ribs.
Cartilage (Joint spaces)	• Assess vertebral endplates to ensure adjacent ones are parallel.
Soft tissues	• Note any soft tissue anomalies.
	• Remember, even though this is an image of the cervical spine, some lung tissue will be present.
Significant areas	• Alteration in height of vertebral bodies can indicate compression fractures.
	• Double lines of spinous process are a sign of clay shoveler's fracture (Fig. 8.9B).
	• Alteration to the alignment of endplates could be a sign of disc herniation.

Anteroposterior Open Mouth

Adequacy

Ensure that all anatomical features are present on the image.

The odontoid process and the atlanto-occipital joint should be clearly visible in the open mouth view.

The inferior surface of the upper central incisors should be superimposed on the occipital bone.

Alignment

The lateral margins of the lateral masses of the 1st cervical vertebral should be aligned with the superior articular process of the 2nd cervical vertebra (Fig. 8.5).

Bones

Review the cortical and trabecular patterns of each individual bone for any disruption, particularly at the odontoid peg. Beware the teeth; the occiput and soft tissue can create appearances that mimic fractures of the odontoid peg.

Cartilage

The distance between the odontoid process and the medial side of the lateral masses of 1st cervical vertebra should be equal (Fig. 8.5) when there is no rotation of the head.

The articular surfaces of the lateral masses of the 1st cervical vertebral and the superior articular facts of the 2nd cervical vertebral should be parallel (Fig. 8.5).

Significant Areas

The odontoid process fracture can be divided into three types (Fig. 8.6). Type I occurs through the tip of the spinous process. Type II occurs where the odontoid process meets the body. Type III occurs through the body of the 2nd cervical vertebra involving the odontoid process.

Misalignment at the lateral masses needs to be noted.

Fig. 8.5 A, Open mouth view of cervical spine. **B,** Lateral alignment of 1st and 2nd cervical vertebrae (yellow lines). Symmetrical joint spaces between articular surfaces (red lines). Equal distance between odontoid process and lateral masses (green lines). (Source: Rosen's Emergency Medicine: Concepts and Clinical Practice, Eighth Edition, 2014.)

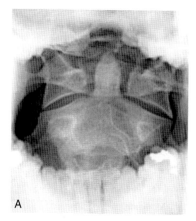 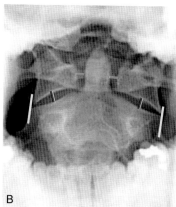

A   B

Systematic Approach

Open mouth view of the cervical spine

Follow the standard approach to the AABCSS in addition to:

Adequacy
- Assess the image for rotation. Rotation of the head will affect the uniformity of the distances between the odontoid process and the lateral masses.
- Ensure all anatomy is included.
- Ensure that the inferior aspect of the incisor teeth and occiput are superimposed.

Alignment
- Lateral alignment of 1st and 2nd cervical vertebra

Bones
- Review the cortical and trabecular patterns of bones following the lines.

Cartilage (Joint spaces)
- Assess distance between the odontoid process and the medial side of the lateral masses of 1st cervical vertebra.
- Assess the articular surfaces of the lateral masses of the 1st cervical vertebra and the superior articular facts of the 2nd cervical vertebra.

Significant areas
- Odontoid process
- Lateral masses

Fig. 8.6 Types of odontoid process fractures. (Redrawn from Anderson LD, D'Alonzo RT: Fractures of the odontoid process of the axis, J Bone Joint Surg Am 56:1663–1674.s, 1974.)

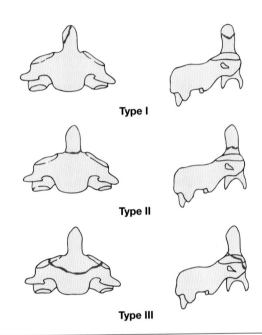

Type I

Type II

Type III

Fractures

The following set of cervical spine images demonstrate disruption to one or more areas described in the above section.

Clinical presentation of cervical spine injuries:

For cervical spine injuries clinical presentation can vary from neck pain through to various degrees of neural deficits, with the most severe being loss of function when the spinal cord is involved. The areas affected will depend on the vertebral level of injury at which the spinal cord is damaged. This will provide some indication as to the level of spinal injury. Fig. 8.7 represents dermatomes of the body. Dermatomes map the body into areas of the skin that are attached to specific nerve segments. Using these as a guide can indicate which vertebral level has been affected.

The following levels of injury identify the function that is lost at various levels along the spinal cord.

 INSIGHT

For the loss of function described at a stated level you need to appreciate that all loss of function for the levels below would also occur.

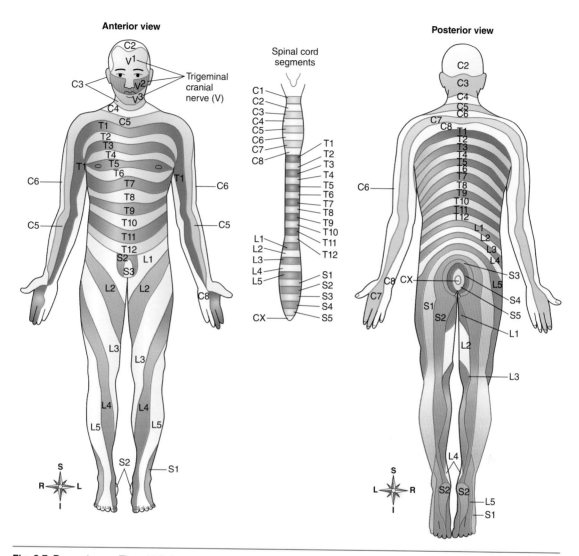

Fig. 8.7 Dermatones. The middle image represents the spinal cord with the nerve segments corresponding to the nerve segments identified on the anterior view (image on the left) and the posterior view (image on the right). (Source: From Patton K, Thibodeau G: The Human Body in Health & Disease, Seventh Edition, St. Louis, 2018, Mosby.)

Damage to:
C3 and above results in a loss of diaphragm function; patients would require artificial ventilation
C4 results in a significant loss of use of biceps and shoulders
C5 results in a loss of the use of wrists and hands
C6 causes the patient to have limited wrist control and there is a loss of hand control
C7 and T1 leads to the patient having some use of their arms but this is limited. Loss at this level is considered to be the threshold for independent living.
T1–T8 results in affected intercostal and abdominal muscles
The lumbar region affects the hips and legs.

Teardrop Fracture

Typical mechanism of injury:

A teardrop fracture can be as a result of a flexion or extension injury. Extension teardrop injuries generally occur higher in the spine, as in Fig. 8.8; usual site is the 2nd cervical vertebra. Flexion teardrop injuries that occur below the 2nd cervical vertebra are considered more severe than extension injuries. Flexion injuries tend to be a result of severe trauma. Extension teardrop injuries tend not to result in neural deficit, as they tend to be stable. Flexion injuries due to the severity are considered unstable and can result in neural deficit.

The common appearance is disruption of the anterior and posterior vertebral lines. In addition to this, there is a triangular piece of bone displaced from the vertebral body anterior. Some of these features can be seen on Fig. 8.8. Clear disruption of the cortical margin of the vertebral body of the 2nd cervical vertebra can be seen.

Fig. 8.8 Teardrop fracture. Disruption of anterior vertebral line and disruption of cortex noted. No evidence of disruption to posterior vertebral line. Reduction in disc space noted inferiorly as an unrelated finding. (Source: Skeletal Trauma: Basic Science, Management, and Reconstruction, Fifth Edition, 2015.)

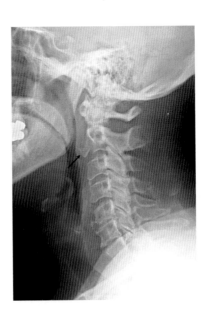

Clay-Shoveler's Fracture

Typical mechanism of injury:

Can occur due to direct force to the spine, as a result of road traffic accident and sudden muscle contraction.

 INSIGHT

Due to the nature of clay digging, the clay would stick to the shovel. This would cause an unexpected force which results in the fracture noted in Fig. 8.9A and B.

Clinical presentation:

These fractures tend to be asymptomatic when they occur and are discovered as incidental findings.

Fig. 8.9 Clay-shoveler fracture. A, note that the fracture of 6th cervical spinous process is the obvious one visualised. On closer inspection there is a second spinous injury present in the 7th cervical spinous process. This represents a good example to continue searching the radiographic image. (Source: Essentials of Radiology, Fourth Edition, 2019.) **B,** green arrow represents the part of the spinous process unaffected. Red arrow represents the fracture part of the spinous process. (Source: Skeletal Imaging: Atlas of the Spine and Extremities, Second Edition, 2011.)

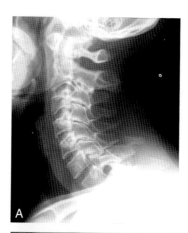

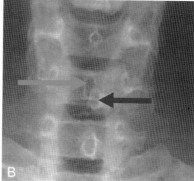

This type of fracture demonstrates the importance of reviewing the spinous process line as it is the spinous process that is fractured, as demonstrated in Fig. 8.9A and B.

Remember that it is important to trace the cortical outlines of all features. In Fig. 8.9B there appear to be 2 radiopaque outlines representing a spinous process. One of the outlines is where you would expect it to be in line with the others, whereas the other one is more lateral. The outline which is in line represents the part of the spinous process that remains attached, whereas the second outline represents the fractured part of the spinous process.

Facet Joint Subluxation and Dislocation

Typical mechanism of injury:

Normally this type of injury is as a result of a flexion force. Rotational forces can be involved when single facets are involved. As with other spinal injuries this can be due to motor vehicle accidents or sports injuries.

Intervertebral facet joints can be subluxated (misaligned) or dislocated. This type of disruption can vary in appearances on the radiographic image: a non-uniform intervertebral facet joint wider at the posterior aspect;

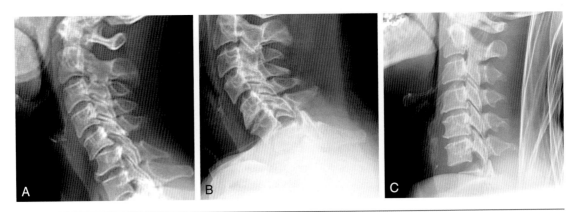

Fig. 8.10 Facet subluxation and dislocation. A represents a facet joint subluxation. Note the widening of the gap between the spinous processes of the 5th and 6th cervical vertebrae. Facet joint at the superior aspect is not comparable to the others. There is also a reduced intervertebral disc space and disruption to the anterior vertebral line. **B** and **C** both represent bilateral dislocations of the facet joints. There are similarities in the disruption of the anterior and posterior vertebral lines. The increased space between the adjacent spinous process and the non-uniformity of the disc space compared to the others. In Fig. 8.9B the disc space has been reduced, whereas in Fig. 8.9C the disc space is increased in size. (Sources: Diagnostic Imaging: Spine, Fourth Edition, 2021.)

the inferior articular facet of the joint being perched on the superior one; complete dislocation. The appearance of other features becomes disrupted, such as the intervertebral disc spaces and an abnormally increased distance between the adjacent spinous processes, as well as disruption of the vertebral lines. Examples of the appearance of this type of injury can be seen in Figs. 8.10A–C.

Hangman's Fracture
Typical mechanism of injury:

This type of fracture is as a result of a hyperextension injury.

The hangman fracture can be difficult to identify if a systematic review is not followed and the cortical outlines of each vertebra are not traced. In Fig. 8.11 there is clear evidence that there is an injury present as noted by the soft tissues swelling present. Upon closer inspection a radiolucent line can be observed between the body of the 2nd cervical vertebra and the pedicles which represents the fracture.

Fractured Odontoid Process
Typical mechanism of injury:

Various mechanisms of injury can cause a fracture of the odontoid process including flexion or extension. In the young the typical cause of injury is a motor vehicle accident, whereas in the elderly the injury is typically caused by falls which involve low energies.

In Fig. 8.12A a fracture of the odontoid process can be seen. There is a disruption of the cortical margin of the body of the 2nd cervical with the odontoid process, and there is a radiolucent line between the body and inferior

Fig. 8.11 Hangman's fracture. (Source: Essentials of Radiology, Fourth Edition, 2019.)

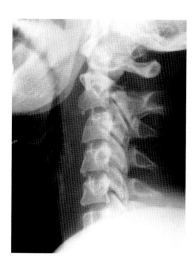

Fig. 8.12 A and B, Type II odontoid process fracture. The fracture is much less clear on the lateral Fig. 8.11B. There is the presence of a radiolucent line between the body and the odontoid process. Note the soft tissues swelling at the area of injury. (Source: Skeletal Trauma: Basic Science, Management, and Reconstruction, Fifth Edition, 2015.)

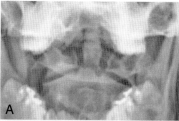

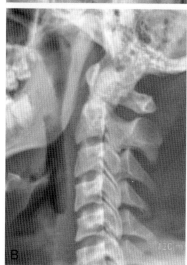

aspect of the odontoid process. The space between the odontoid process and the lateral masses is not uniform. These appearances are consistent with a type II odontoid process fracture (Fig. 8.6).

Jefferson's Fracture (Burst Fracture)

Typical mechanism of injury:

Diving head-first into shallow water; this results in compression loading causing the 1st cervical vertebra to fracture.

This type of fracture is visualised through the non-alignment of the lateral masses with the lateral aspect of the body of the 2nd cervical vertebra (Fig. 8.13). It also demonstrates the limitations of the radiographic image, as this type of fracture results in more than one fracture involving both the anterior and posterior arches that are not visualised. Asymmetry around the odontoid process can occur, as well as widening of the gap between the odontoid process and the lateral masses.

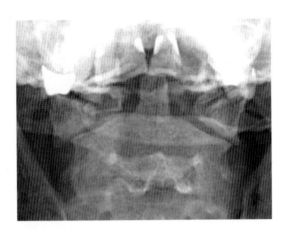

Fig. 8.13 Jefferson's fracture. Note the non-alignment laterally and the widened distance between the odontoid process and the lateral masses. (Source: Learning Radiology: Recognizing the Basics, Second Edition, 2012.)

 INSIGHT

When checking for symmetry, first check the technical quality of the image to ensure that the patient is not rotated. Rotation of the patient's head will result in loss of symmetry and an unequal distance between the odontoid process and lateral masses.

INSIGHT

Remember to check all aspects of the image and not just focus on the cervical spine.

From the potential impact on the patient due to majority of the cervical spine injuries, it can be appreciated why computed tomography is a modality of choice. This allows the full extent of the injury to be appreciated, which can be difficult to appreciate from radiographic imaging.

THORACIC SPINE

 INSIGHT

The thoracic spine is the transition between the cervical and lumbar spine. As such, the thoracic vertebrae change in size, being smaller at the cervical end to larger at the lumbar end.

Lateral

Adequacy

Ensure that all anatomical features are present on the image.
 The shoulders obscure the vertebra at the upper end of the thoracic spine.

Alignment

These lines should all follow a normal kyphotic curve representing a primary curvature of the thoracic spine. Normal curvature of the thoracic spine is between 20° and 40°.

Anterior Vertebral Line
This line is located at the anterior aspects of the vertebral bodies and should be a smooth uninterrupted line (Fig. 8.14B).

Posterior Vertebral Line
This line is located at the posterior aspects of the vertebral bodies and should be a smooth uninterrupted line (Fig. 8.14B).

Fig. 8.14 A and B, Lateral thoracic spine. Note how the size of the vertebral bodies increases from the superior to the inferior aspect. This is also the case for the vertebral disc spaces. **B,** Anterior vertebral line (red). Posterior vertebral line (green). (Sources: Merrill's Atlas of Radiographic Positioning & Procedures, Fifteenth Edition, 2023.)

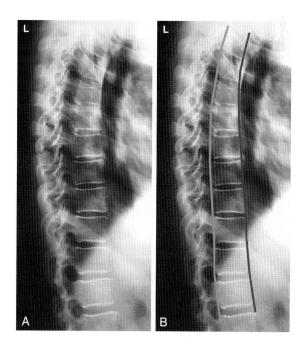

Due to increase in size of the vertebral bodies from the superior to inferior, the lines diverge. To take this into account, ensure that you assess the alignment of each corner of vertebral body at the level above with the one at the level below.

Bones

Review each vertebra, taking note of the vertebral body, pedicle, articular processes, and spinous process (Fig. 8.14). The vertebral bodies increase in size as they transition from the cervical to the lumbar region.

Cartilage

The intervertebral disc spaces will increase in size from the superior to inferior.

Systematic Approach

Lateral view of the thoracic spine
Follow the standard approach to the AABCSS in addition to:

Adequacy	• Ensure all anatomy is included. • Ensure that the image is lateral.
Alignment	• Use lines and follow these to note any disruption to one or more lines.
Bones	• Review the cortical and trabecular patterns of bones following the lines. • Review the vertebral bodies. Remember, they increase in size from superior to inferior.
Cartilage (Joint spaces)	• The intervertebral discs increase in height from cervical to lumbar region.
Significant areas	• Note change in shape to vertebral bodies. This area is a common area to be affected by collapse and wedge fractures.

Anteroposterior

Adequacy

Ensure that all anatomical features are present on the image from thoracic vertebra 1 to 12.

Alignment

Spinous Process
The spinous process should form a central line.

Vertebral Bodies
Should be aligned. The vertebral bodies increase in size from the cervical to the lumbar region.

Pedicles
The pedicles form two straight lines on either side of the spinous process towards the lateral margins of the vertebral bodies. The distance between the pedicles increases from superior to inferior, resulting in the lines diverging.

Bones

Vertebral bodies gradually increase in size from superior to inferior aspects. Review each vertebra, taking note of the cortical margins of vertebral body, pedicle, articular processes, and transverse and spinous processes.

Assess whether there is any loss in height of the vertebral bodies.

The pedicles appear as ovals at the superolateral aspect of the vertebral bodies. They are often referred to as the eyes of the vertebrae.

Assess the ribs that are included as well as the clavicles.

Fig. 8.15 A and B, Anteroposterior thoracic spine view. **B,** The green line represents spinous process alignment; the blue oval encloses a pedicle; the red lines demonstrate the superior and inferior vertebral endplates representing a uniform intervertebral disc space. (Source: Bontrager's Textbook of Radiographic Positioning and Related Anatomy, Tenth Edition, 2021.)

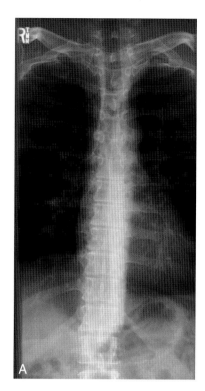
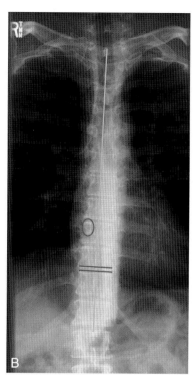

 INSIGHT

On the anteroposterior image the natural kyphosis of the thoracic spine can result in differential magnification, giving the appearance of increased size of vertebra towards the superior and inferior aspects of the image.

Cartilage (Fig. 8.15)   Each intervertebral disc space should be uniform in height across the two vertebral bodies it is situated between. To assess this, review the superior and inferior vertebral endplates; they should be parallel.

Soft Tissue   Paraspinal lines (also known as paravertebral, paraspinous lines or stripes), Fig. 8.17A and B.

These lines are adjacent to the vertebral bodies, and in normal circumstances the right is not visualised when there is no abnormality; aspects of the left may be visualised. In cases where there is associated pathology, the paraspinal lines can become visible and will be accentuated (Fig. 8.17C and D). One cause of raised paraspinal lines is a haematoma in the region where there is a vertebral fracture.

INSIGHT

A fracture may not be visible on the anteroposterior view, but the deformity of the paraspinal line would indicate that there is an abnormality present.

Systematic Approach

Anteroposterior view of the thoracic spine
Follow the standard approach to the AABCSS in addition to:

Adequacy	• Ensure all anatomy is included. • Ensure that there is no rotation.
Alignment	• Ensure spinous processes are aligned. • Ensure alignment of vertebral bodies.
Bones	• Review the cortical and trabecular patterns of bones. • Review vertebral bodies for any loss in height. • Review pedicles.
Cartilage (Joint spaces)	• Assess that each individual intervertebral disc space is uniform.
Soft tissues	• Assess the paravertebral lines for any increase.
Significant areas	• Vertebral bodies as a result of compression injuries.

Fractures

Compression Fracture

Clinical presentation:

Patients can be asymptomatic. Back pain is one presentation. If there are numerous compression fractures, as in the case of patients suffering from severe osteoporosis, the patient will present with a greater degree of kyphosis.

Typical mechanism of injury:

Fall from a height, motor vehicle accident, and actions resulting in hyperflexion forces.

Look for changes in the size of the vertebral bodies. Reduction in the height of the anterior aspect of the vertebral body compared with another vertebra demonstrates a collapsed vertebra (Fig. 8.16).

Fig. 8.16 Compression fracture. (Source: Cecil Essentials of Medicine, Tenth Edition, 2022.)

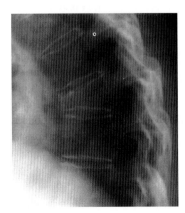

INSIGHT

The vertebrae have a large amount of trabecular bone present to help maintain their integrity. Trabecular bone has a faster turnover than cortical bone and will be affected early by factors that affect bone turnover, for example, the menopause. This in will reduce the integrity of the bones, with the forces of gravity acting to make them susceptible to wedge fractures/collapse.

Figs. 8.17 Paraspinal lines. **A** and **B** represent normal paraspinal line appearances, the left one being visualised, using the yellow dotted line, whilst the right one is not. **C** and **D** represent raised left and right paraspinal lines (red dotted lines). Note the loss of height of one of the vertebrae at the site of the raised paraspinal lines. (Sources: Radiología de urgencias y emergencias, Tercera edición, 2015.)

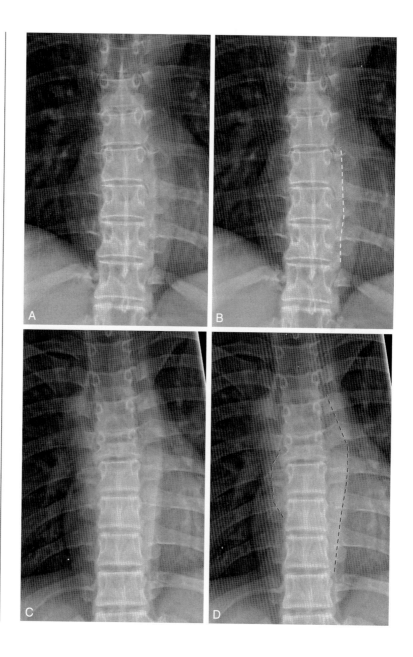

Raised Paraspinal Lines

Clinical presentation:

Back pain

Typical mechanism of injury:

Any mechanism of injury resulting in a fracture of the vertebral body.

Remember, even when there is no apparent disruption to the bony anatomy, there can be soft tissue evidence that there is an injury present. Fig. 8.17 C and D demonstrates raised paraspinal lines, indicating an injury is present. Raised paraspinal lines are a result of a haematoma (Fig. 8.18).

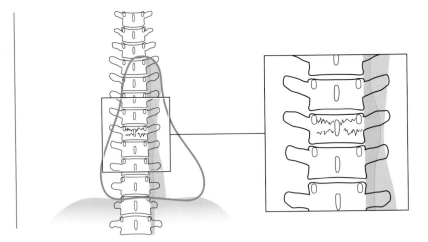

Fig. 8.18 Diagrammatic representation of the presence of vertebral haematoma resulting in raised left paraspinal line. (Source: Accident & Emergency Radiology: A Survival Guide, Second Edition, 2005.)

LUMBAR SPINE

Lateral

Adequacy   Ensure that all anatomical features are present on the image, including the spinous processes and the thoracolumbar junction to the sacrum.

Alignment

Anterior Vertebral Line
This line is located at the anterior aspects of the vertebral bodies and should be a smooth uninterrupted line (Fig. 8.19B).

Posterior Vertebral Line
This line is located at the posterior aspects of the vertebral bodies and should be a smooth uninterrupted line (Fig. 8.19B).

These lines should all follow a normal curve lordosis representing the secondary curvature of the lumbar spine. Normal curvature of the lumbar spine is between 40° and 60°.

Bones

Review the cortical outline of each individual vertebra.

Vertebral bodies should be 'square' and of equal height (Fig. 8.19C), with the exception of 5th lumbar vertebra, which is deeper anterior than posterior.

Endplates between adjacent vertebrae are parallel (Fig. 8.19)

Cartilage

Intervertebral disc spaces increase in size from those between the 1st and 2nd lumbar vertebrae (L1/L2) to those between the 4th and 5th lumbar vertebrae (L4/L5). The intervertbral disc between the 5th lumbar vertebra and the 1st sacral segment (L5/S1) is usually narrower (Fig. 8.19).

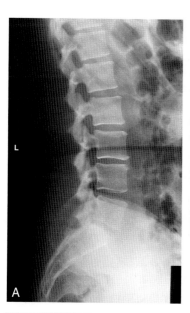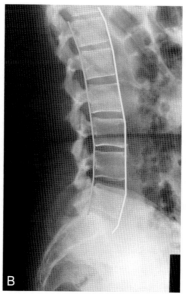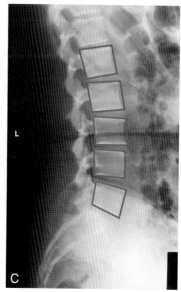

Fig. 8.19 A–C Lateral lumbar spine. B demonstrates the anterior (yellow) and posterior vertebral lines (green). Note that the inferior and superior end plates are parallel. **C** represents the square shapes of the vertebra. Note how the size in the intervertebral disc changes. (Source: Merrill's Atlas of Radiographic Positioning & Procedures, Fifteenth Edition, 2023.)

Review the facet joints.

Lateral view of the lumbar spine

Follow the standard approach to the AABCSS in addition to:

Adequacy
- Ensure all anatomy is included.
- Ensure that the image is lateral.

Alignment
- Use lines and follow these to note any disruption to one or more lines.

Bones
- Review the cortical and trabecular patterns of bones following the lines.
- With the exception of the 5th lumbar vertebra, all others should be of equal height and square.

Cartilage (Joint spaces)
- The vertebral disc height increases in size up to L5/S1, which is narrower.
- Facet joints should be reviewed.

Significant areas
- Assess the size of vertebral bodies; these can become wedged or biconcaved.
- Assess the pedicles and spinous process for any disruptions.

Anteroposterior

Adequacy

Ensure that all anatomical features are present on the image and include the T11/T12 junction to the Sacrum and sacroiliac joints

Alignment

There is a smooth continuous lateral outline on both sides of the vertebral bodies.

Assess alignment of the spinous processes; these should be central in the vertebral body if there is no rotation (Fig. 8.20A and B).

The distance between pedicles (interpedicular distance) increases from the 1st to the 5th lumbar vertebrae (Fig. 8.20A and B). The pedicles create two diverging lines. If a pair of pedicles do not follow this pattern, this is indicative of an injury.

Bones

The vertebral bodies are 'square' and of equal height (Fig. 8.20A and B).

The distance between adjacent spinous processes is fairly uniform (Fig. 8.20A and B).

Pedicles are visualised on both sides and on all the lumbar vertebrae and are oval.

All transverse processes of the lumbar spine are visualised, and there is no disruption to the cortical margins (Fig. 8.20A and B).

Assess the ribs, thoracic vertebrae, and sacrum.

Cartilage

Superior and inferior endplates between adjacent vertebrae are parallel. Intervertebral disc spaces tend to increase from L1/L2 to L4/L5. L5/S1 is usually narrower. This is difficult to appreciate on the AP image due to angle of spine and diverging beam.

Sacro-iliac joints are of equal width.

Soft Tissues

Ensure the psoas muscle shadows are visible (Fig. 8.20A and B).

No alteration to soft tissue noted lateral to the vertebral bodies.

Fig. 8.20 A and **B,** The blue line represents the alignment of the spinous processes. The green dashed lines are the outlines of the psoas muscles. The yellow double arrows demonstrate the distance between the pedicles. (Source: Merrill's Atlas of Radiographic Positioning & Procedures, Fifteenth Edition, 2023.)

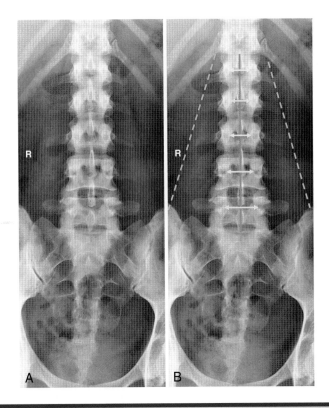

 INSIGHT

Due to the lordotic angulation of the lumbar spine and the divergence of the X-ray beam, visualisation of the lower disc spaces is difficult to assess.

Anteroposterior view of the lumbar spine
Follow the standard approach to the AABCSS in addition to:

Adequacy	• Ensure all anatomy is included • Ensure that there is no rotation
Alignment	• Review alignment of the vertebral bodies • Review alignment of spinous processes • Review interpedicular distance
Bones	• Review the cortical and trabecular patterns of each bone following the lines • Note any disruption to the transverse processes • Ensure both pedicles are visible
Cartilage (Joint spaces)	• The intervertebral disc height increases in height to L5/S1, which is narrower. • Assess symmetry of sacroiliac joints.
Soft tissues	• Note any soft tissue anomalies.
Significant areas	• Size of vertebral body, height is lost when there is a compression fracture. • Widening of pedicles • Transverse processed

Fractures

Clinical presentation of lumbar spine injuries:

Back pain (mid, lower) and/or neurological deficits of the lower limbs and lower bodily functions.

Compression Fracture

These can also be known as wedge fractures and crush fractures.

Typical mechanism of injury:

Fall from a height, motor vehicle accident, and actions resulting in hyperflexion forces (Fig. 8.21 and Fig. 8.22).

Fig. 8.21 Demonstrates a compression fracture following a vertical force after jumping from a roof. These is a reduction in anterior height of the first lumbar vertebral body compared with the rest, indicating a compression fracture. Note the disruption to the anterior vertebral line. There is disruption noted to the cortical margin to the 1st lumbar, indicating fracture to the vertebral body. (Source: Emergency Radiology: The Requisites, 2009.)

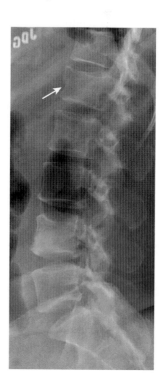

Burst Fracture

Typical mechanism of injury:

This type of fracture is as a high-energy force along the axial axis of the body, which is not too dissimilar to the Jefferson's fracture described earlier. Common causes are motor vehicle accidents and falls from a significant height, with the person tending to land on their feet.

Fig. 8.23 represents both the anteroposterior and lateral views demonstrating a burst fracture. On the anteroposterior view the changes can be noted on the affected vertebra. The changes of note are the change in shape of the vertebra. The affected vertebra appears wider and the lateral margins of its body are not congruent with those of the bodies of the superior and inferior vertebrae. The height of the vertebral body also appears reduced. The key feature is the

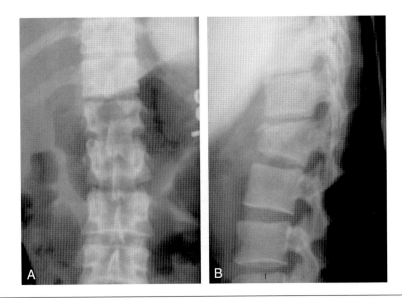

Fig. 8.22 Demonstrates a compression fracture following hyperflexion. A, Anteroposterior view of the lumbar spine. Note the loss of height of the 1st lumbar vertebral body. In addition to this there is also a fracture of the left transverse process. The increased distance between the spinous process of the 12th thoracic vertebra and 1st lumbar vertebra indicates that the mechanism of injury was hyperflexion. **B,** Lateral view of the lumbar spine. Note the loss of height to the anterior aspects of the 1st lumbar vertebral body. (Source: Skeletal Trauma: Basic Science, Management, and Reconstruction, Fourth Edition, 2009.)

Fig. 8.23 Anteroposterior and lateral views of the lumbar spine demonstrating a burst fracture. (Source: Imaging Skeletal Trauma, Fourth Edition, 2015.)

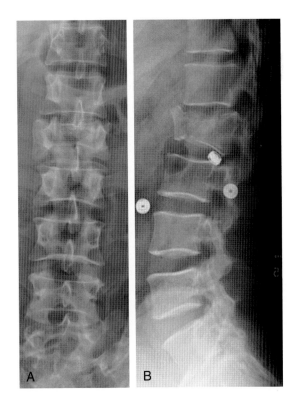

distance between the pedicles. The distance between the pedicles of the affected vertebra is wider than that of the inferior pedicles, which is not normal. This indicates that the vertebral foramen has been disrupted.

On the lateral image disruption is noted to both the anterior and posterior vertebral lines. There is disruption to the cortical margin of the affected lumbar vertebra. The body of the vertebra has lost its square shape and appears wedged. From the lateral perspective the appearance is not too dissimilar to the compression fracture described previously.

Chance Fracture

Typical mechanism of injury:

This type of injury occurs as a result of hyperflexion. The most common cause described is a motor vehicle accident where the individual is wearing a lap seat belt, although falls from heights have also been cited as a cause.

Fig. 8.24A and B demonstrate a Chance fracture at the level of the 2nd lumbar vertebra. Fig. 8.24A, the lateral view, demonstrates the typical appearance of a Chance fracture. There is wedging of the 2nd vertebral body and a horizontal line noted through the pedicles and pars interarticularis. This image does not demonstrate the full extent of the injury due to the spinous processes having not been included on the image. Had the spinous process been included, then the fracture of the spinous process would have been noted, which is demonstrated on Fig. 8.24B.

Fig. 8.24B demonstrates a horizontal radiolucent line running through the body of the 2nd lumbar vertebra. On closer inspection the radiolucent line passes through the inferior aspect of both pedicles and the upper part of the spinous process, creating discontinuity of these features. This discontinuity further supports the findings demonstrated on the lateral image and confirms the fracture of the spinous process. There is some loss of the height of the vertebral body of the 2nd lumbar vertebra.

Fig. 8.24 A and **B,** Lateral and anteroposterior views of the lumbar spine demonstrating a Chance fracture of the 2nd lumbar vertebra. **C** 3D computed tomography (CT) reconstruction of 2nd lumbar vertebra demonstrating the extent of the injury through the spinous process. (Source: Imagerie des traumatismes rachidiens, 2007.)

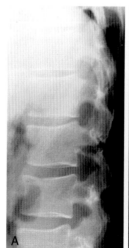
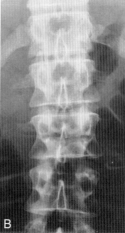
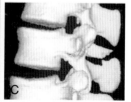

INSIGHT

A Chance fracture can result in an empty vertebral body sign. Due to the posterior displacement of structures, they no longer are superimposed on the vertebral body, and as such, the vertebral body appears empty of features on an anteroposterior view.

CONCLUSION

The descriptions in this chapter are one approach to interpreting radiographic images of the spine. There are other similar approaches, for example, the ABCDE method, where the letters represent the following aspects: A = alignment, B = bodies, C = cortical outline, D = disk spaces, E = edges, and soft tissue. This method covers the same aspects described in this chapter. The most important thing is to use whichever method works for you in order for you to undertake a thorough review of the radiographic image, ensuring that no aspect is overlooked.

A number of examples in this chapter use only one view to demonstrate the change. The key aspect of viewing radiographic images is the assimilation of information from all the images. Review all the radiographic images to establish whether the changes being noted are supported by the full series of images. In addition to this you should now appreciate the complexity of demonstrating spinal injuries on radiographic images. In several examples used the full extent of the injury cannot be established from the radiographic image and hence the move to other imaging modalities in this case CT being the first line of examination in major trauma involving the spine.

Further Reading

Atlas, S. W., Regenbogen, V., Rogers, L. F., & Kwang, K. S. (1986). The radiographic characterization of burst fractures of the spine. *AJR Am J Roentgenol, 147*(3), 575–582.

Pal, D., Sell, P., & Grevitt, M. (2011). Type II odontoid fractures in the elderly: an evidence-based narrative review of management. *Eur Spine J, 20*, 195–204. doi:10.1007/s00586-010-1507-6.

Walter, J., Doris, P. E., & Shaffer, M. A. (1984). Clinical presentation of patients with acute cervical spine injury. *Ann. Emerg. Med., 13*(7), 512–515.

FACIAL BONES

9

Facial bones are formed by a collection of irregularly shaped bones. Some of these bones are extremely delicate, and injury to these may not be visualised on radiographic imaging. The overlapping of anatomical features on radiographic images of the facial bones makes reviewing the images complex. It is important that you have a good understanding of the anatomical features present and how these are demonstrated in order to appreciate what is being visualised on radiographic images. As with any other axial skeletal anatomy, key principles when considering the radiographic image are symmetry, alignment, and shapes.

FACIAL BONES

For all projections check the cortical margins of each bone. This is complex with facial bones due to the numerous overlapping features present causing overlying shadows. In addition to this, the delicate nature of some of the bones makes it difficult to ascertain whether there is an injury present.

Check for disruption of the trabecular bone patterns.

There may be indications of injury that may not be visualised, for example, fluid in the sinuses or soft tissue signs.

 INSIGHT

Facial bones are delicate, and a fracture can be difficult to detect. Due to the complexity of anatomy and the potential difficulty in identifying injury in some cases, facial bone radiographic imaging examinations are becoming less common and are being replaced by computed tomography.

OCCIPITOMENTAL (WATERS VIEW)

Adequacy

Ensuring the patient is not rotated is essential. There are a number of ways this can be achieved. One way is to assess whether the distance between the lateral aspect of the skull and the lateral margin of the frontal process on each side is equidistant. By ensuring that the patient is not rotated symmetry can be used to assess the radiographic image by comparing the left and right sides to note any changes.

The petrous ridges should be below the maxillary sinuses. This ensures that any radiopacities present in the maxillary sinus are not obscured by the petrous ridges.

 INSIGHT

It is common for fluid levels to be present due to the blood in a maxillary sinus as an indication of injury.

Alignment

There are various lines that can be used. The following is a modification of the McGrigor-Campbell lines (Fig. 9.1B). All lines should be undisrupted.

Supraorbital line: extends from the frontozygomatic sutures across the superior margin of both orbits and frontozygomatic suture of the opposite side.

Infraorbital line: extends from the superior aspect of one zygomatic arch, along the infraorbital margin, across the nasal bone, and along the infraorbital margin and superior aspect of the zygomatic arch of the opposite side.

Inferior zygomatic line: extends from the inferior aspect of the zygomatic arch, along the lateral margin of the maxillary antrum, across the maxillary alveolar margin, and then along the lateral margin of the maxillary antrum and inferior aspect of the zygomatic arch of the opposite side.

Superior mandibular line: extends from the mandibular condyle along the mandibular notch and coronoid process and follows the alveolar margins and along the coronoid process, mandibular notch, and mandibular condyle of the opposite side.

Inferior mandibular line: extends from the mandibular condyle, down the mandibular ramus, to angle of the mandible along the inferior border of the body of the mandible to the symphysis menti, then follows these aspects on the opposite side.

These lines follow known areas where fractures can occur.

Bones

Review the cortical and trabecular patterns of bones following the lines above, searching for any disruption. There are numerous lines present that represent the overlying shadows of the structures of the facial bones and skull.

Cartilage

It is important to assess the temporomandibular joints. These are included as part of the mandibular. The condyle of the mandible is a location where fractures can occur.

Assessing the sutures is important, as identified in Chapter 3; a suture is an area that is more susceptible to damage due to not being as strong as bone.

Soft Tissues

Review the radiographic image for any soft tissue swelling. Free air may be present in the superior aspect of the orbit; this is as a result of air entering the orbital cavity from a fracture involving a sinus. The appearance is of a radiolucent crescent below the supraorbital margin. A blowout fracture involves the delicate bones of the orbit. As a result of the fracture, soft tissue from the orbit may be seen in the superior aspect of the maxillary sinus below the infraorbital margin resulting in a radiopacity. Check for any foreign bodies.

Significant Areas

The lines described in alignment follow the significant areas where injuries occur.

Systematic Approach   Radiographic appearances of the facial bones (Fig. 9.1B)

Occipitomental (Waters view)
Follow the standard approach to the AABCSS in addition to:

Adequacy	• Assess the image for rotation • The petrous ridges should be below the maxillary sinuses.
Alignment	• Use a recognised set of lines and follow these to ensure that you assess the image fully.
Bones	• Review the cortical and trabecular patterns of bones following the lines.
Cartilage (Joint spaces)	• Assess the temporomandibular joints • Assess the sutures
Soft tissues	• Note any soft tissue swelling • Review the sinuses for any radiopacity and radiolucency

Fig. 9.1 A, Occipitomental projection. **B,** Occipitomental projection modified McGrigor-Campbell lines: 1 represents the supraorbital line; 2 represents the infraorbital line; 3 represents the inferior zygomatic line: 4 represents the superior mandibular line; 5 represents the inferior mandibular line. (Source: Musculoskeletal Trauma: A Guide to Assessment and Diagnosis, 2011.)

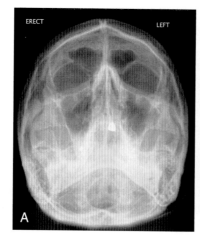 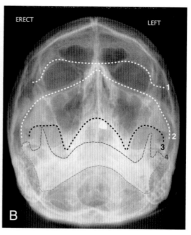

Significant areas • Check the appropriate line for the following:
  - widening of the sutures
  - black eyebrow sign
  - zygomatic arch
  - inferior rim of orbits
  - nasoethmoid and medial orbits
  - maxillary alveolar margins
  - condyle of mandible
  - coronoid process
  - alveolar margins of the mandible
  - ramus of the mandible
  - angle of the mandible
  - body of the mandible

OCCIPITOMENTAL 30° VIEW

Adequacy

Ensuring the patient is not rotated is essential. There are a number of ways this can be achieved. One way is to assess if the distance between the lateral aspect of the skull and the lateral margin of the frontal process on each side is equidistant. By ensuring that the patient is not rotated symmetry can be used to assess the radiographic image by comparing the left and right sides to note any changes.

Due to the use of a 30° caudal angle, this projection is more tangential and allows better appreciation of the lower orbital margin. On this projection it is easier to discern whether there is anterior or posterior disruption of the lower orbital margin. The zygomatic arches and the lateral walls maxillary antra are also well demonstrated.

 INSIGHT

Due to the 30° caudal angulation of the beam, fluid levels will not be visualised. Fluid levels can only be visualised when a horizontal X-ray beam is used. Consider a glass half filled with water. Looking at the glass from above, the air is above the water, and therefore the distinction between the air and the water cannot be appreciated. This is akin to using a vertical X-ray beam. Now look at the glass from the side: the distinction between the water and the air can be seen as a fluid level, and this is the same principle as when a horizontal X-ray beam is used.

Alignment

The same assessment for alignment as previously described for the occipitomental view can be used. The following is a modification of Campbell lines (Fig. 9.2B). All lines are curves and should be undisrupted.

Line 1: extends from the frontozygomatic sutures across the superior margin of both orbits and frontozygomatic suture of the opposite side.

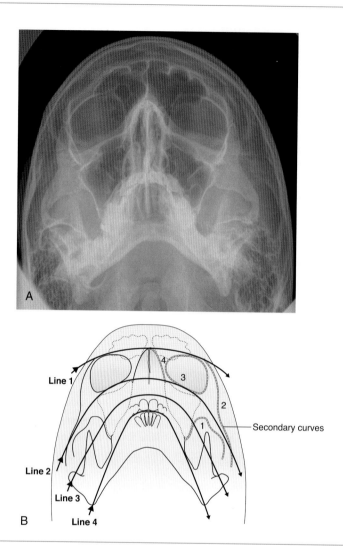

Fig. 9.2 Occipitomental 30°. A, Radiographic image of occipitomental 30°. **B,** Diagrammatic representation of occipitomental 30° demonstrating Campbell lines. (Source: Essentials of Dental Radiography and Radiology, Sixth Edition, 2021.)

Line 2: extends from the zygomatic arch, along the infraorbital margin, across the nasal complex, and along the infraorbital margin and zygomatic arch of the opposite side.

Line 3: extends from the mandibular condyle, through the coronoid process, lateral aspect of maxilla, across the base of the nasal complex, then through the lateral aspect of the maxilla, to traverse the coronoid process and finish at the mandibular condyle of the opposite side.

Line 4: extents from the angle of the mandible through the alveolar margins of the mandible to the angle of the mandible of the opposite side.

Bones

Review the cortical and trabecular patterns of bones following the lines above, searching for any disruption.

Cartilage

As for the occipitomental it is important to assess the temporomandibular joints, as is assessing the sutures.

Soft Tissues

Review the image for any soft tissue swelling. Check for any foreign bodies.

Significant Areas

The lines described in alignment follow the significant areas where injuries occur.

Systematic Approach Radiographic appearances of the facial bones (Fig. 9.2A and B)

Occipitomental 30°
Follow the standard approach to the AABCSS in addition to:

Adequacy	• Assess the image for rotation. • Good visualisation of the lower orbital margins, zygomatic arches, and lateral walls maxillary antra.
Alignment	• Use a recognised set of lines and follow these to ensure that you assess the image fully.
Bones	• Review the cortical and trabecular patterns of bones following the lines.
Cartilage (Joint spaces)	• Assess the temporomandibular joints. • Assess the sutures.
Soft tissues	• Note any soft tissue swelling. • Review the sinuses for any radiopacity and radiolucency.

Significant areas	• Check the appropriate line for the following:
	  • widening of the sutures
	  • zygomatic arch
	  • inferior rim of orbits
	  • nasoethmoid and medial orbits
	  • maxillary alveolar margins
	  • condyle of mandible
	  • coronoid process
	  • alveolar margins of the mandible
	  • ramus of the mandible
	  • angle of the mandible
	  • body of the mandible

ORTHOPANTOMOGRAM (OPT/OPG)

Adequacy

As the examination uses a moving X-ray beam and image detector, the image takes a short time to acquire and there is the possibility of movement unsharpness. Assess the image to determine whether there is any blurring due to movement unsharpness. If the patient is not correctly positioned, there is the possibility that the mandible and teeth are not sharp and in focus; this too results in blurring. As with the occipitomental and occipitomental 30°, ensure there is symmetry. Fig. 9.3 demonstrates the typical appearance of an orthopantomogram image.

Fig. 9.3 Orthopantomogram. (Source: BASICS Mund-, Kiefer- und Plastische Gesichtschirurgie, 2016, [P132].)

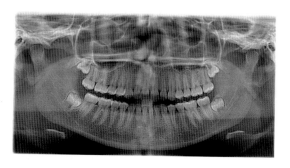

 INSIGHT

The nature of the injury may result in the disruption of symmetry.

Alignment

Use appropriate lines to follow the superior and inferior aspects of the mandible. Do not forget to review other anatomy present on the image.

Superior mandibular line: extends from the mandibular condyle along the mandibular notch and coronoid process and follows the alveolar margins and along the coronoid process, mandibular notch, and mandibular condyle of the opposite side.

Inferior mandibular line: extends from the mandibular condyle, down the mandibular ramus, to angle of the mandible along the inferior border of the body of the mandible to the symphysis menti, then follows these aspects on the opposite side.

Bones

Review the cortical and trabecular patterns of bones following the lines above, searching for any disruption.

Cartilage

As for the orthopantomogram, it is important to assess the temporomandibular joints.

Soft Tissues

Review the image for any soft tissue swelling. Note that there are numerous soft tissues shadows present that can be confusing.

Significant Areas

The lines described in alignment follow the significant areas where injuries occur. Fig. 9.10 is a diagrammatic representation of common areas where injuries to the mandible can occur.

Orthopantomogram (OPT/OPG)
Follow the standard approach to the AABCSS in addition to:

Adequacy	• Ensure there is no blurring due to movement unsharpness. • Ensure that the mandible and teeth are sharp and in focus. • There is symmetry (Fig. 9.3).
Alignment	• Use a recognised set of lines and follow these to ensure that you assess the image fully.
Bones	• Review the cortical and trabecular patterns of bones following the lines.
Cartilage (Joint spaces)	• Assess the temporomandibular joints.
Soft tissues	• Be aware of soft tissue shadows.

Significant areas	• Check the appropriate line for the following:
	  • condyle of mandible
	  • coronoid process
	  • alveolar margins of the mandible
	  • ramus of the mandible
	  • angle of the mandible
	  • body of the mandible
	• Check all teeth.
	• Assess maxillary sinuses for radiopacities.

 INSIGHT

Be aware that the site of impact may not be the site of fracture. Due to the shape of the mandible, the force of the impact will be transferred to the opposite side and can thus cause a fracture of the side opposite to the impact. This type of injury is known as a contracoup.

The mandible can be considered a U-shaped structure; as such, if a fracture is noted, be aware that a second fracture may be present. But it is not uncommon for single fractures to exist.

Fractures

Fractures can occur in numerous places. Areas where facial fractures can occur are the frontal bone, the nasal bones, zygomaticomaxillary region, orbital region, mid-face, and mandible.

Typical mechanism of injury:

A direct hit to the zygoma. As can be seen in Fig. 9.4, there are a number of sutures associated with the zygoma.

Clinical presentation:

Tenderness, bruising, and swelling over the zygoma.

These fractures commonly involve the zygomatic arch, inferior orbital rim, walls of the maxillary sinus, and lateral orbital wall (Fig. 9.4A–E). The following sutures may or may not be involved: temporozygomatic, zygomaticomaxillary, frontozygomatic, and sphenozygomatic (Fig. 9.4D). This type of fracture has been referred to as tripod, tetrapod, quadripod, malar, or trimalar fracture. Common reasons for the occurrence of this type of injury are following: assault, a road traffic accident, or a fall.

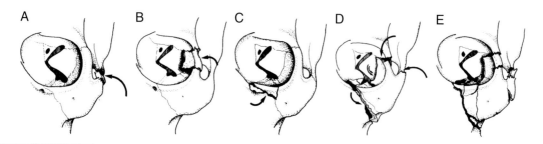

Fig. 9.4 A dsssiagrammatic representation of various types of zygomaticomaxillary complex fracture. **A,** represents a single fracture to the zygomatic arch. **B,** represents a fracture only affecting the lateral orbital wall. **C,** represents a fracture to the infraorbital margin. **D,** represents a fracture through the temporozygomatic, zygomaticomaxillary, frontozygomatic, and sphenozygomatic sutures. **E,** represents multiple fractures through the zygomaticomaxillary complex fracture. (Source: Zingg M, Laedrach K, Chen J, et al.: Classification and treatment of zygomatic fractures: a review of 1025 cases. J Oral Maxillofac Surg 50:778, 1992.)

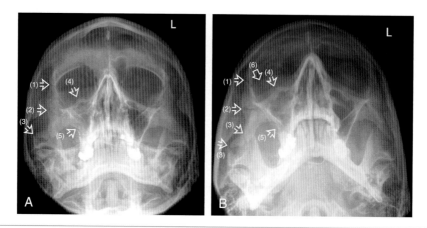

Fig. 9.5 A and B, Zygomaticomaxillary complex fracture. The arrows denote the areas that have been disrupted. *Alignment:* The supraorbital, infraorbital, and inferior zygomatic lines have all been disrupted. Comparing symmetry it is noted, particularly on image **B,** the occipitomental 30°, that there is a radiolucent line in the region of the right frontozygomatic suture (1). There is a radiolucent noted at the lateral margin of the right orbit (2). The smooth line of the right zygomatic arch has been disrupted (3). The line of the inferior orbital margin on the right has been disrupted (4). The lateral margin of the right maxillary antrum has a radiolucent line (5). *Bones:* Disruption to cortical margins can be seen throughout the images (2), (3), and (5). *Soft tissue:* Swelling can be noted at the lower orbital margin on the right. Note that the increase in radiopacity in the right maxillary sinus is indicative of a presence of increased density. (Source: Essentials of Dental Radiography and Radiology, Sixth Edition, 2021.)

Fig. 9.6 Zygomaticomaxillary complex fracture.
Alignment: The infraorbital and inferior zygomatic lines have all been disrupted at the right zygomatic arch.
Bones: Clear disruption to the cortical margins of the right zygomatic arch.
(Source: Essential Surgery: Problems, Diagnosis and Management, Sixth Edition, 2020.)

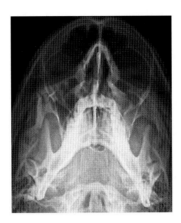

 INSIGHT

The use of the prefix 'tri-' in the description of these fractures can be a misnomer, as they frequently involve four components.

Radiographic appearance:
The radiographic appearance of these fractures can vary. Figs. 9.4–9.6 demonstrate some of the locations of the fracture and some typical radiological appearances.

Le Fort Fractures

Midface fractures are classed as Le Fort. There are three types of classification, all involving the separation of the facial bones from the bones of the cranium (Fig. 9.7). Le Fort type I fracture is horizontally through both maxillae. The upper teeth are separated from the rest of the face. Le Fort type II fractures are through both maxillae and through nasofrontal suture, having a triangular appearance. In Le Fort type III the fracture line separates the cranial bones from the facial bones, whereas the other two types involve fractures of the facial bones. Low-velocity facial injuries tend to be associated with Le Fort type I fractures, whereas high-velocity injuries are associated with Le Fort type II and III fractures.

Between 10 and 20% of facial injuries are a type of Le Fort fracture.

Typical mechanism of injury:
Le Fort injuries are associated with sports, particularly football, hockey, and baseball. Road traffic accidents also can result in Le Fort injuries.

Le Fort type I fractures are as a result of a direct blow to the upper teeth. The direction of the blow is in downwards direction.

Le Fort type II fractures are as a result of a blow to the lower or mid-maxillary region.

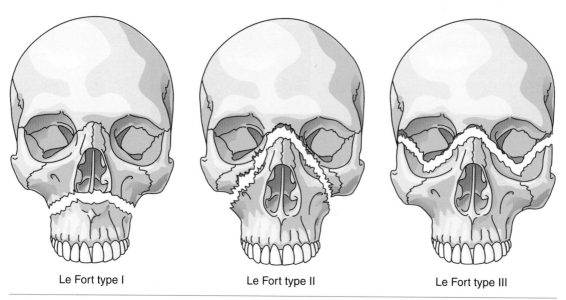

Le Fort type I   Le Fort type II   Le Fort type III

Fig. 9.7 Le Fort fractures. (Source: Good VS, Kirkwood: Advanced Critical Care Nursing, Second Edition, St. Louis, 2018, Elsevier.)

Le Fort type III fractures are as a result of a blow to the upper maxillary region at the junction of the nasal and frontal bones.
Clinical presentation:

Le Fort type I:
Bruising around the injury site with swelling of the upper lip. Due to disruption of the maxilla, the upper teeth are misaligned with the lower teeth.

Fig. 9.8 Le Fort type I.
Alignment: Disruption to the supraorbital and infrazygomatic lines is noted. Widening of the frontozygomatic suture is noted on the left side when symmetry is compared along the supraorbital line. The signs of the Le Fort I fracture are noted with the bilateral disruption of the infrazygomatic line at the regions lateral borders of the maxillary antra. *Bones:* radiolucent line caused by disruption of the cortical margins of lateral borders of the maxillary antra. (Source: Textbook of Oral Radiology, Second Edition, 2015.)

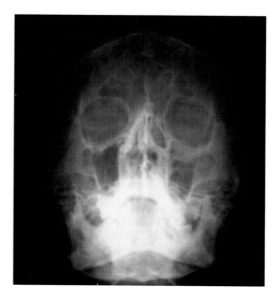

Le Fort type II:

The clinical presentation is the same as for the Le Fort type I fracture with significant deformity and swelling. There is swelling and bruising around the eyes, as well as bleeding from the nose. One deformity is the widening of the space where the upper and lower eyelids meet. The maxilla and nose are movable due to the lack of attachment of the bones with the rest of the face.

Fig. 9.9 Le Fort type II.
Alignment: Disruption to infraorbital and infra zygomatic lines. *Bones:* Radiolucent lines are noted bilaterally through the cortical bone margins of the lateral walls of both maxillary sinuses. There is also bilateral disruption of the cortical margins of the lower orbital floor that also present as radiolucent lines. The signs of injury are consistent with the patterns noted for a Le Fort II injury. The fracture across the nose is not visualised. (Source: Radiographie et radiologie dentaires, 2019.)

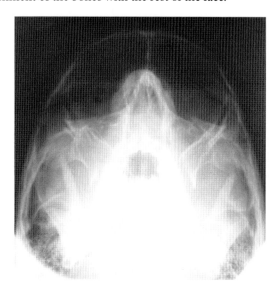

Le Fort type III:

Like the Le Fort type II injury, there is swelling and bruising around the eyes, as well as facial deformity. The separation of the facial bones from the rest of the cranium results in an increased length of the face that is also flattened. Compared to the other types, there is more extensive bruising. There is also cerebrospinal fluid discharge from the ear and nose as well as blood in the middle ear.

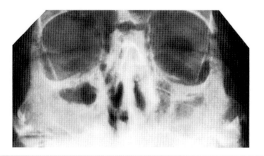

Fig. 9.10 Le Fort type II and III. *Alignment:* Disruption to supraorbital, infraorbital, and infrazygomatic lines. *Bones:* Radiolucent lines are noted bilaterally through the frontozygomatic sutures. A radiolucent line is noted across the frontonasal and frontomaxillary sutures. These disruptions are representative of a Le Fort III injury. In addition to these features, there is also bilateral disruption of the cortical margins of the lower orbital floor that also presents as radiolucent lines. This would be consistent with the a Le Fort II injury, although disruption to the maxillary bones is not noted. There is also bilateral injury noted to the zygomatic arch. *Soft tissue:* A fluid collection can be noted in the right maxillary sinus, with the left maxillary sinus appearing opaque. (Source: Grainger & Allison's Diagnostic Radiology: A Textbook of Medical Imaging, 2014.)

Mandibular Fractures

Typical mechanism of injury:

   Mandibular fractures can occur all along the mandible, as can be seen in Fig. 9.11. There are various causes of mandibular fractures, such as road traffic accidents, fights, assaults, accidents including falls, and being kicked by an animal.

Clinical presentation:

   Mandibular fracture can cause malocclusion. There is bruising at the site of injury and soft tissue swelling. The teeth may be damaged and could be loose. Nerves could be affected, and there may be a loss of sensation. Depending on whether the fracture is stable or not, it may result in increased mobility of the mandible in cases of instability.

Fig. 9.11 Classification of mandibular fractures. (Source: Core Procedures in Plastic Surgery, 2014.)

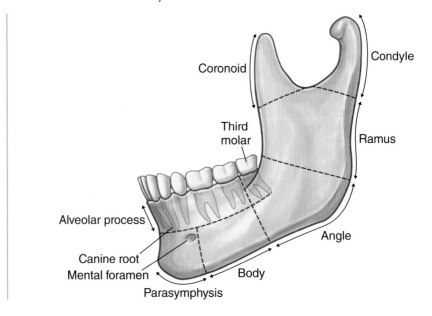

Condyle and body

Fig. 9.12 Orthopanto-mogram demonstrating a fractured left condyle and right body. *Alignment:* Both the supramandibular and inframandibular lines are disrupted at the left condylar region and right body. *Bones:* Cortical disruption can be noted in the condylar region and body. In the region of the body radiolucent lines are present. (Source: Oral and Maxillofacial Surgery, Second Edition, 2009.)

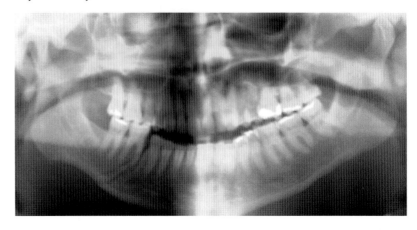

Parasymphysis and angle

Fig. 9.13 Orthopanto-mogram demonstrating fractures in the regions of the right parasymphysis and left angle. *Alignment:* Both the supramandibular and inframandibular lines are disrupted at the right region of the parasymphysis and the left angle. *Bones:* Cortical disruption can be noted in the right region of the parasymphysis and the left region of the angle, with the presence of radiolucent lines in both regions. At the region of the right parasymphysis a clear step in the bone is visible. (Source: McMinn's Color Atlas of Head and Neck Anatomy, Fifth Edition, 2017.)

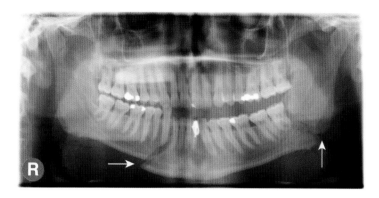

Soft Tissue

There are specific soft tissue signs that are indicative of a fracture. These are opacities in the ethmoid and maxillary sinuses. In the maxillary sinuses an opacity in the superior aspect of the antrum below the infraorbital margin is associated with a blowout fracture known as a teardrop sign. This can have an accompanying thin plate of bone present in the maxillary antrum. A fluid line in the inferior aspect of the maxillary antrum can be indicative of the presence of blood. The presence of air in the superior aspect of the orbit is known as a black eyebrow sign. Fig. 9.14 is a diagrammatic representation of where these signs can be located.

 INSIGHT

For the black eyebrow sign and the fluid level in the maxillary antrum to be visible, the patient needs to be erect, as the air will rise and fluid will descend due to gravity. Fluid levels will be visualised when a horizontal X-ray beam is employed.

Fig. 9.14 Soft tissue signs. 1, teardrop sign. 2, fluid level in maxillary antrum. 3, bone fragment in maxillary antrum. 4, black eyebrow sign. 5, opacity in ethmoid sinus. (Source: Accident & Emergency Radiology: A Survival Guide, Second Edition, 2005.)

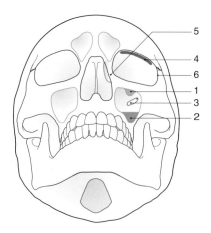

Teardrop sign as a result of orbital floor fracture

Typical mechanism of injury:

Force placed on the orbit in Fig. 9.15A from a punch to the orbit will result in compression of the orbit. Other causes of an orbital floor fracture include falls and road traffic accidents. The thin bone of the inferior aspect of the orbit will fracture, hence the presence of fragments of bone Fig. 9.15B. In addition to this, vessels in the bone will be disrupted, causing blood to enter and collect in the maxillary antrum and form a fluid level. Tissue at the inferior aspect of the orbit will be suspended in the maxillary antrum forming a teardrop sign (Fig. 9.15B).

Clinical presentation:

The eye may not be in its normal position due to the increased space created by the fracture. The patient may be suffering from double vision and swelling around the eye. If the sinus is involved, then air may be present, resulting in the black eyebrow sign (see below for details). There may be loss of sensation over the zygoma.

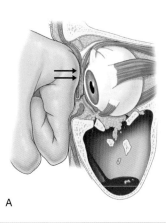

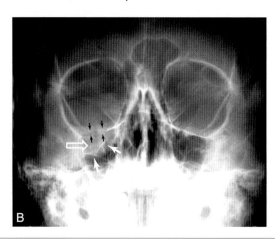

Fig. 9.15 Teardrop sign as a result of a blowout fracture. A, demonstrates the force and resultant damage caused. **B,** *Alignment:* Demonstrates disruption to infraorbital margin line. *Bones:* Discontinuation of the infraorbital cortical margin as denoted by the black arrows. Fragments of bone noted in maxillary antrum white arrows. The soft tissue of the teardrop sign is noted suspended from the infraorbital margin, as identified by the white arrow outline. (Sources: Neligan P, Buck D, eds: Core Procedures in Plastic Surgery, Philadelphia, 2014, Elsevier; Essentials of Radiology, Fourth Edition, 2018.)

Black eyebrow sign as a result of frontal bone fracture

Fig. 9.16 Black eyebrow sign. *Alignment:* Disruption to supraorbital line. *Bones:* disruption noted to cortical right superior orbital margin, with associated radiolucent line. *Soft tissue:* crescent-shaped radiolucency noted at the superior aspect of the right orbit representing the black eyebrow sign. (Source: Musculoskeletal Trauma: A Guide to Assessment and Diagnosis, 2011.)

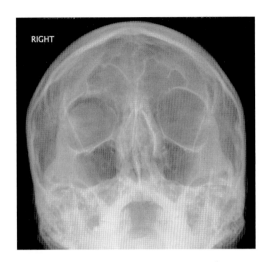

Fluid level

Various methods of injury described in this chapter can result in the disruption of bone and the collection of blood in the maxillary sinus.

Fig. 9.17 Fluid level, left sinus. *Adequacy:* The interpretation of this image is limited by the presence of the superior margin of the petrous ridge (solid white arrow). This could obscure fluid if it was not above the petrous ridge, as is the case on the left side (outline white arrow). (Source: McMinn's Color Atlas of Head and Neck Anatomy, Fifth Edition, 2017.)

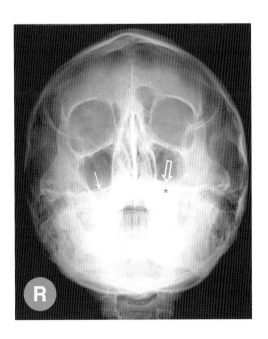

CONCLUSION

As can be seen from this chapter, facial bones are complex and can be difficult to review. Following a systematic approach can help in identifying any sign of injury and ensuring that you trace outlines of bones and assess the image for symmetry. Where there is asymmetry, ask yourself the question: is this due to rotation or is there an abnormality present?

Further Reading

Hopper, R. A., Salemy, S., & Sze, R. W. (2006). Diagnosis of midface fractures with CT: What the surgeon needs to know. *RadioGraphics;, 26*, 783–793. doi:10.1148/rg.263045710. Published online.

Kane, M., Tamba, B., Gassama, C. B., Diatta, M., Ba, A., Kounta, A., Boucaid, A. M., Kebe, N. F., & Tine, S. D. (2021). Clinical and radiological aspects of mandibular fractures: A review of 128 cases. *International Journal of Oral Health Dentistry, 7*(4), 282–286. https://www.ipinnovative.com/open-access-journals.

Koenen, L., & Waseem, M. (2021). *Orbital Floor Fracture.* StatPearls Publishing LLC. Bookshelf ID: NBK534825PMID: 30521246.

Laine, F. J., Conway, W. F., & Laskin, D. M (1993). Radiology of maxillofacial trauma. *Current Problem in Diagnostic Radiology, 22*(4), 145–188. doi:10.1016/0363-0188(93)90019-p.

Patel, B. C., Wright, T., & Waseem, M. (2021). *Le Fort Fractures.* StatPearls Publishing LLC. Bookshelf ID: NBK-526060PMID: 30252316.

Pickrell, B. B., Serebrakian, A. T., & Maricevich, R. S. (2017). Mandible fractures. *Seminars in Plastic Surgery, 31*(2), PMC5423793.

Susarla, S. M., & Peacock, Z. S. (2014). Zygomaticomaxillary complex fracture. *ePlasty, 14*: ic27.

PRACTICAL APPLICATIONS OF IMAGE INTERPRETATION AND THE FUTURE 10

Throughout this book we have focused on how to approach image interpretation of the musculoskeletal system. It is essential that medical images are correctly interpreted in order that the patients receive an accurate diagnosis and appropriate treatment, and that resources are maximised. Errors occur in image interpretation, and it is essential that these errors are minimised. There is evidence that demonstrates that multiple appropriately educated observers improve image interpretation. By following a systematic approach and increasing your knowledge and understanding of the subject of image interpretation you can improve your ability in this area. This book acts as a starter along your journey, and other texts, resources, education, and training will help you further develop your skills in this area.

WHAT IS THE BENEFIT OF MORE INDIVIDUALS BEING ABLE TO INTERPRET MEDICAL IMAGES ACCURATELY?

With an increased workload for radiologists, reduction in radiologists, and the advancement of imaging modalities and technology procedures there are insufficient radiologists to undertake all the reporting necessary. This necessitates ways in which other professions can help reduce the burden whilst ensuring that there is no deterioration in service.

METHODS EMPLOYED IN IMAGE INTERPRETATION

Image interpretation can be used in different ways in the clinical environment. One system that can be used is flagging that there is an abnormality present, commonly referred to as the 'red dot' system or radiographer abnormality detection system (RADS). Historically the flagging occurred through the attachment of a red dot sticker to the image and more recently the addition of a 'red dot' annotation on digital images. This method allows the radiographer to indicate that they have identified an abnormal feature on the image via the application of an agreed-upon flagging system. This method is of benefit in cases where the referrer is a member of staff who has limited experience in image interpretation and can aid in reducing errors.

The main flaw of this approach is the lack of specificity regarding how many injuries are present and what has been identified on the image to the referrer. The referrer is made aware that potential abnormality has been detected but not the exact location or frequency. Over-reliance on the system may mean that when no flag is used, an assumption is made that there is no abnormality. It could be the case that an abnormality has been overlooked or the individual has decided not to indicate that they have identified an abnormality. For this method to be effective it is essential that all participate in the system to prevent confusion of the referrer in cases where a flag has not been applied. This method is the most commonly employed in the trauma setting. There is evidence that education improves an individual's ability in this area.

An advancement on the 'red dot' system is 'preliminary clinical evaluation'. This incorporates a written statement identifying where the abnormality has been identified, thus reducing the potential for ambiguity as identified by the 'red dot' system. The communication of findings, as well as the inability to provide a preliminary clinical evaluation, must be communicated to avoid confusion. Key to this approach is the use of appropriate language that is understood by all and is unambiguous. The systematic approach to image interpretation described through the chapters of this book is a starting point providing you with areas to review in order to aid you in recognising changes. You need to appreciate that this book is not a comprehensive coverage of all injuries but provides examples of how the systematic approach applies to the various anatomical regions covered. This approach can be synthesised and applied to new patterns you encounter in order to appreciate the changes present. You can consider this as a form of detective model, as identified in Chapter 1, where you are gathering evidence from the image to reach your conclusion. Utilising this approach means that you are able to justify your decision if required.

What, Where, and How

The What, Where, and How method can be employed to help you focus on the main aspects of what needs to be included in your final comment on the image. Reviewing your evidence using this approach to answer each aspect (What, Where, and How) allows you to break down the components of the injury, developing an understanding of what is present on the radiographic image in order to communicate your findings unambiguously to other professionals so as to answer the clinical question asked in the imaging request and identify any other significant finding(s) observed.

The What Aspect Relates to Considering

What is hindering you from interpreting the radiographic image? Consider *adequacy*: is there anything that does not allow you to fully assess the image, e.g. artefacts, non-standard projection due to patient immobility, or other limitations?

What is the abnormality? Fracture/dislocation/subluxation/*soft tissue* sign

What is the appearance? Is it radiopaque/radiolucent line, the direction of the line

The Where Aspect Relates to Considering

Where is the abnormality located? This can be subdivided into:

Where in the body? Which *bones* are involved, are *joints (cartilage)* involved, is it intra-articular/extra-articular?

Where on the bone? Proximal/mid/distal

Where within the bone? Diaphysis/metaphysis/epiphysis/*Significant areas* (anatomical feature, e.g. tuberosity)

The How Aspect Relates to Considering

How does the injury appear? Displaced/angled *alignment*

How is the structure displaced/angled? Consider direction of displacement of the fracture: posterior/anterior; medially/laterally; distally/proximally

How much displacement is there? Minimally to grossly

 INSIGHT

The extent of displacement can be controversial, as image interpretation is idiosyncratic. Remember, it is an art, and the appreciation of art, by its nature, is a personal thing. In extreme cases, for example, when there is gross displacement, a judgement can be easily made and you do not need years of education and knowledge to recognise the radiographic appearance. The decision becomes much more complex when you are considering the distinction between normal and minimal displacement, as we have seen in Chapter 3, Fig. 3.16A. Other difficulties in judging displacement are at boundaries. What is the threshold between minimal and mild; mild and moderate; and moderate and severe? Fig. 10.1 is an adaptation from Robinson (1997) which attempts to identify which cases can be considered easier and which more difficult. As you can see, this system is not perfect and leaves itself open to personal interpretation.

Fig. 10.1 Threshold of easy and difficult cases. (Source: Robinson P: Radiology's Achilles' heel: error and variation in the interpretation of Röntgen images, Br J Radiol 70(839):1085–1098, 1997.)

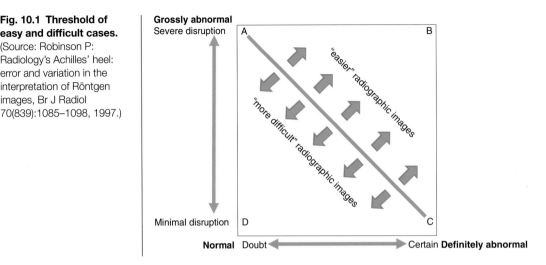

The vertical (Y) axis in Fig. 10.1 represents the range of radiographic images from normal, where there may be minimal disruption which can be difficult to distinguish from normal, to grossly abnormal, where there is severe disruption to anatomy present on the radiographic image, whereas the horizontal (X) axis ranges from radiographic images that have normal appearances to those that have definitely abnormal appearances. The diagonal line from the letter 'A' to 'C' is a threshold, where radiographic images above the line can be considered 'easier' to identify as being abnormal and those below the line as 'more difficult'. At point D, where there might be a minimal disruption, you may not be confident that what you are observing is an abnormality, but it may be a pattern on the radiographic image that is giving the impression of an injury, and this will raise doubt due to your lack of confidence in your observation, whereas at the opposite extreme at point B you can be certain that there is an injury due to severe disruption present. This can be used to explain why normal images take longer to view and interpret than those where the injury is obvious.

Audit

A key aspect of any individual involved in radiographic image interpretation is quality assurance, and this can be achieved through audit. You can review your work against the final report to identify areas of discrepancy. Any discrepancies can be identified and recommendations can be made with a SMART (Specific, Measurable, Achievable, Realistic, and Time-related) action plan. Audit should be viewed as a method to improve and can be applied as a learning aid for all the systems identified above. Fig. 10.2 is one that you could use integrating the various aspects covered throughout this book to help develop your ability in radiographic image interpretation.

Fig. 10.2 Proposed model for audit.

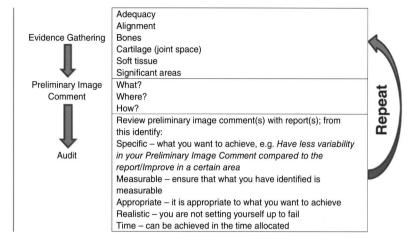

Evidence Gathering	Adequacy Alignment Bones Cartilage (joint space) Soft tissue Significant areas
Preliminary Image Comment	What? Where? How?
Audit	Review preliminary image comment(s) with report(s); from this identify: Specific – what you want to achieve, e.g. *Have less variability in your Preliminary Image Comment compared to the report/Improve in a certain area* Measurable – ensure that what you have identified is measurable Appropriate – it is appropriate to what you want to achieve Realistic – you are not setting yourself up to fail Time – can be achieved in the time allocated

Repeat

Eponyms

One reason for discrepancy could be the use of eponyms. Through the What, Where, and How approach the focus is on summarising the findings and describing what changes are present, whereas the report could use eponyms and acronyms, which are a form of shorthand. In this case an eponym is a type of injury that is named after an individual who is associated with the pattern of injury. Throughout chapters of this book eponyms have been used, such as Colles fracture, Salter-Harris classification, and Le Fort type injuries. To establish whether you have accurately described the injury, you have to understand what the pattern of injury the eponym refers to. The scope of this book does not allow for the inclusion of all the eponyms; the suggested further readings section at the end of this chapter includes a paper on eponyms. For eponyms to be useful the user and the referrer must have an understanding of the eponym. A lack of consistency in the use of eponyms can result in miscommunication, and it could be argued that the use of a descriptive highlighting of the noted changes is less likely to cause miscommunication.

 INSIGHT

The eponym Le Fort is named after Rene Le Fort, who was a French surgeon. Facial trauma was caused on cadavers by dropping cannon balls on the face or hitting the face with a bat. Results of the injuries caused by these activities were reviewed, and the types of injuries classified, by Le Fort.

Insignificant Finding

Another reason that there may be a discrepancy between your preliminary image comment and that of the report of an expert is that the changes you have identified are insignificant findings. An insignificant finding is one that does not affect the patient's treatment or management.

EXERCISE

Using Fig. 10.3, radiographic images of a dorsiplantar foot and oblique, undertake an audit following the model in Fig. 10.2. You can compare your answer on page 310.

Fig. 10.3 Dorsiplantar foot and oblique. (Source: JINJ, ISSN 0020-1383, 2010.)

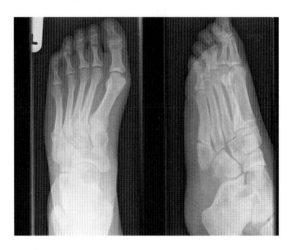

ARTIFICIAL INTELLIGENCE

Throughout the book we have covered observational changes, which have limitations, relying on our visual perception abilities. Other imaging modalities, for example, computed tomography, can rely on measurements to assess size of structures as well as shades of grey related to the Hounsfield unit, which is specific to tissue types. As such, the reporter has more information and evidence on which to base their report. We must recognise that we can only base our decision on the current state of knowledge; in the future, through research and other applications, for example, artificial intelligence (AI), we will be able to gather more information to assist us in reaching a conclusion on radiographic images.

Currently much work is being undertaken with regards to AI in terms of how it could assist in the interpretation of medical images, in addition to other aspects of radiology. AI has already infiltrated many aspects of our life: you may unlock your mobile phone with facial recognition software, you may use smart home devices, you may use satellite navigation while travelling, and cars are equipped with adaptive cruise control, automatic braking, and lane recognition. Your devices can gather information about you so that you can be targeted with recommendations for purchases.

INSIGHT

What is AI?

In simple terms, AI can be considered any task undertaken by a computer which would require human intelligence.

THE BASICS OF AI

AI uses algorithms, which are a set of rules required to be followed by calculation in order to reach solutions. In the case of image interpretation, the solution could be identifying a specific pathology.

Machine learning can be considered as new learning undertaken by the computer based on pre-existing algorithms. Deep learning is a branch of machine learning where algorithms use layers of neural networks that are employed between the input and output to reach a conclusion. In Fig. 10.4 an input, which in this case can be considered as data from a radiographic image, enters the input layer. The data from the radiographic image pass through a series of hidden layers, referred to as the neural network. In each layer aspects will be evaluated according to the algorithm. Once the data have passed through the hidden layers of the neural network and been analysed, it will reach the output layer and provide a response, which would be the findings for the data of the radiographic image in question.

It is predicted that AI will outperform humans in the future. Rather than seeing this as a threat, we need to view this as an opportunity for us to learn from AI and improve our performance. There is the potential for AI to identify patterns that we are currently unaware of or are not distinguishable on a

Fig. 10.4 Artificial neural network. (Source: Biofuels and Bioenergy: Opportunities and Challenges, 2022.)

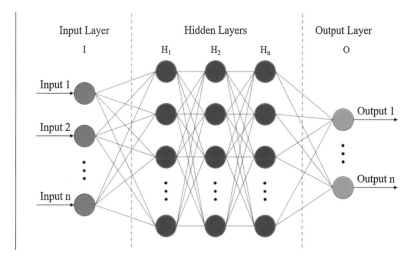

radiographic image when we use vision alone. The data set of the radiographic image may contain imperceptible changes to the eye due to the interaction of the X-ray as it passes through tissue. The analysis of this data is known as radiomics. These subtle changes may be meaninful and in the future be used to aid in the decision making process of an image. It is essential that we adapt and evolve to develop our roles and use the advancements of technology to benefit the patient.

One fear with AI with respect to image interpretation is the lack of understanding of how the algorithms work to reach an output. This potentially has consequences legally if an incorrect conclusion is reached that impacts the patient's diagnosis and treatment.

 INSIGHT

A question that you may ask is: with the evidence that AI is outperforming humans, why do we need to understand image interpretation? We need to understand how AI reaches its conclusion to appreciate what information is being used to reach a decision. This will help us better understand whether other factors can be used to aid us in reaching a decision. In addition to this, we can also have confidence in that decision, as we appreciate how it has been arrived at.

CONCLUSION

Throughout this book we have taken you on a journey to appreciate various factors involved in image interpretation, to appreciate the appearances of injuries on the bones and soft tissue of the musculoskeletal system. You need to recognise that this is the start of your journey with regards to understanding the radiographic image. The application of the systematic approach and audit of your work will help you to recognise your limitation and thus appreciate what you need to do to develop. Any individual involved in image interpretation must ensure that there is a clear scope of practice so that there is a clear understanding of expectations and boundaries, and ensure that they work within these. We see this book as a foundation on which you will develop through further education and clinical experience to reach your potential in this field.

 EXERCISE. ANSWER

Adequacy
Partial left anatomical marker noted on dorsoplantar (DP) view. No anatomical mark noted on dorsiplantar oblique view.
All relevant anatomy included on dorsiplantar and dorsiplantar oblique image.
Adequate density and contrast noted on both images.

Alignment
On DP view no disruption to alignment noted.

On the DP oblique view the width of the fracture would indicate that there is minimal displacement dorsally.

Bones

Cortical margin of fifth metatarsal disrupted at the proximal diaphysis. Transverse radiolucent line noted on the DP view. The diaphysis at the distal aspect to the fracture site of the fifth metatarsal appears expanded at the lateral aspect.

Oblique radiolucent line noted on the DP oblique image. The radiolucent line is wider at the plantar aspect than at the dorsal aspect. At both the proximal and distal aspects of the fracture site the bone appears more radiopaque (sclerotic).

Cartilage (Joint Space)

No disruption noted to joints

Soft Tissue

Soft tissue swelling noted on dorsiplantar image at sight of disruption

Significant Areas

Proximal aspect of the diaphysis of the fifth metatarsal.

What?

Oblique fracture (Why oblique on the DP? There appears to be a radiopacity distal to the radiolucency, which would indicate that bone is overlapping), evidence of fracture healing (sclerotic area and expanded diaphysis)

Where?

Proximal aspect of the diaphysis of the fifth metatarsal

How?

Minimal dorsal displacement.

Preliminary image evaluation:

Oblique fracture of the proximal diaphysis of the fifth metatarsal with minimal dorsal displacement. Evidence is that the fracture is not acute.

Or

Eponym

Jones fracture Torg type III. Evidence is that the fracture is not acute.

You would need to understand the Torg classification system.

Review preliminary image comment(s) with report(s); from this identify:

Specific – what you want to achieve, e.g. *Have less variability in your Preliminary Image Comment compared to the report/Improve in a certain area*

Measurable – ensure that what you have identified is measurable

Appropriate – it is appropriate to what you want to achieve

Realistic – you are not setting yourself up to fail

Time – can be achieved in the time allocated

Further Reading

Bowes, J., & Buckley, R. (2016). Fifth metatarsal fracture and current treatment. *World Journal of Orthopedics, 7*(12), 793–800.

Chetlen, A. L., Chan, T. L., Ballard, D. H., Frigini, L. A., Hildebrand, A., Kim, S., Brian, J. M., Krupinski, E. A., & Ganeshan, D. (2019). Addressing burnout in radiologists. *Acad Radiol, 26*, 526533.

Hargreaves, J., & Mackay, S. (2003). The accuracy of the red dot system can it improve with training? *Radiography, 9*, 283–289.

Hunter, T. B., Peltier, L. F., & Lund, P. J. (2000). Radiologic history exhibit 1 Musculoskeletal eponyms: Who are those guys? *Radiographics, 20*, 828.

Robinson, P. (1997). Radiology's Achilles' heel: Error and variation in the interpretation of Röntgen images. *Br J Radiol, 70*(839), 1085–1098.

Stevens, B., & Thompson, J. (2018). The impact of focused training on abnormality and provision of accurate preliminary clinical evaluation in newly qualified radiographers. *Radiography, 24*, 47–51.

Woznitza, N., Steele, R., Groombridge, H., Compton, E., Gower, S., Hussain, A., Norman, H., O'Brien, A., & Robertson, K. (2021). Clinical reporting of radiographs by radiographers: Policy and practice guidance for regional imaging networks. *Radiography, 27*, 645–649.

INDEX

Note: Page number followed by *f* and *t* indicates figure and table respectively.